Preface

This volume represents the proceedings of the Sapporo International Seminar on Trophoblastic Diseases, held July 13–14, 1985. The theme of this seminar was "Trophoblastic Diseases—Basic and Clinical Approaches."

Advances in medicine as well as in society in general have made human longevity a remarkable feature of recent years. However, various problems facing us in the social and health sciences are interfering with the spread of new medical knowledge. In fact, although progress in the management and treatment of young patients with trophoblastic diseases has improved survival of patients in developed countries, this reduced case fatality is not shared equally among patients in developing countries. The incidence of trophoblastic diseases is high in developing countries. The Sapporo International Seminar was particularly worthwhile in this regard, because it provided a successful forum for fruitful discussions of basic and clinical aspects of trophoblastic diseases by participants from various countries. This publication of the proceedings will inform others of the seminar's achievements.

This volume consists of 19 scientific papers presented at the seminar. As the title implies, the content's cover almost all fields concerning trophoblastic diseases. Half of the papers are purely basic, and others describe the management and the treatment of trophoblastic diseases. Discussions of the papers were especially spirited.

We hope that this book will help medical doctors and students in the field of gynecologic oncology, and researchers in basic science.

Kihyoe Ichinoe, M.D.

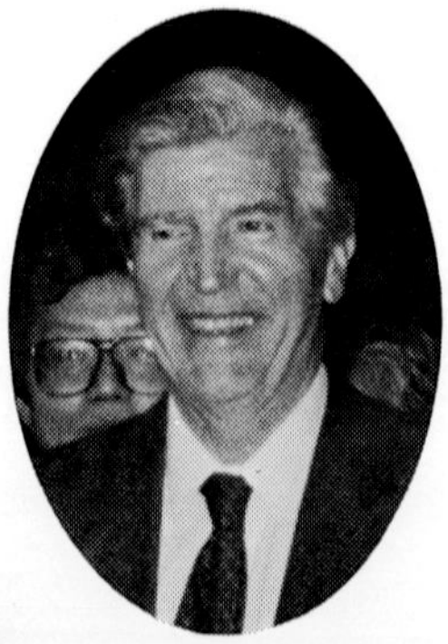

Dr. K. D. Bagshawe

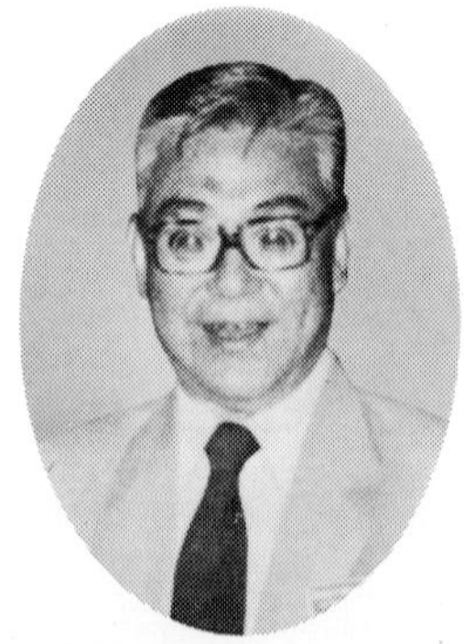

Dr. H. Z. Song

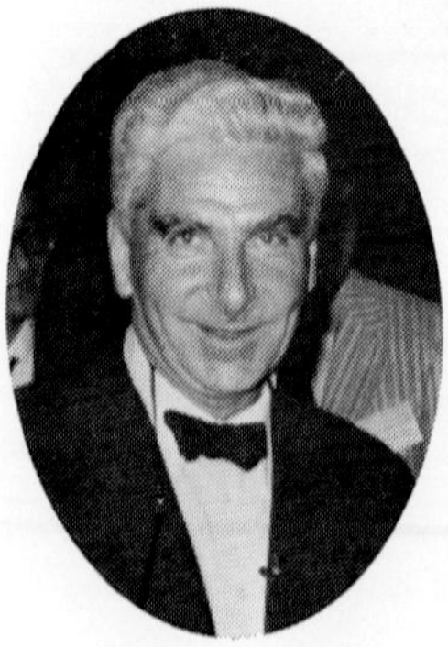

Dr. E. I. Kohorn

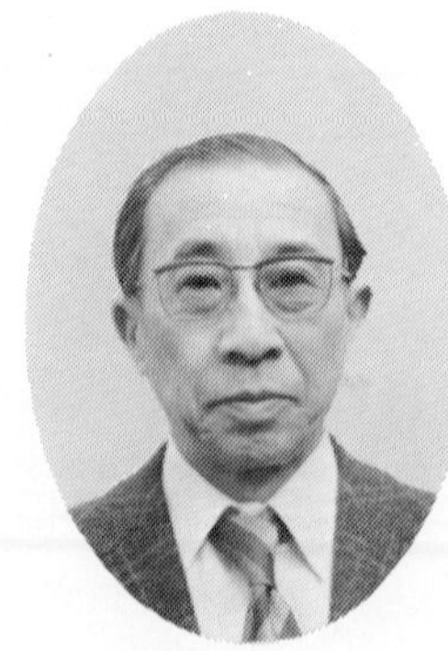

Dr. H. Soma

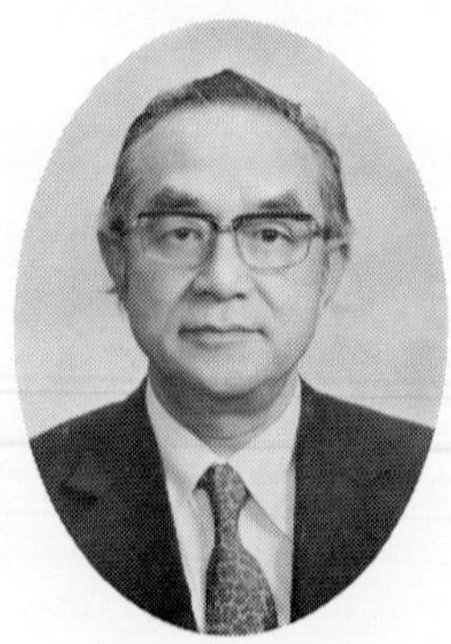

Dr. K. Ichinoe

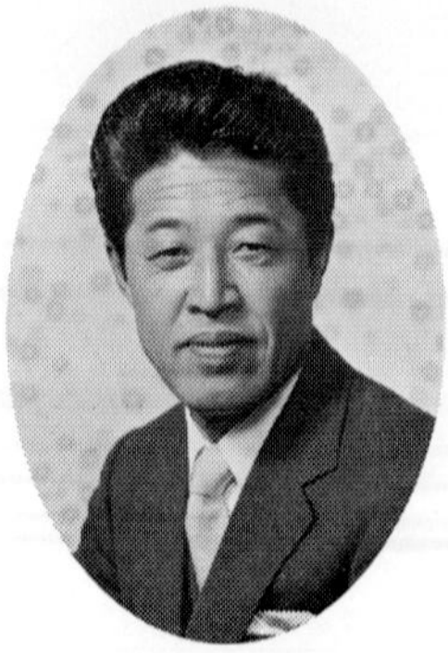

Dr. T. Sugawa

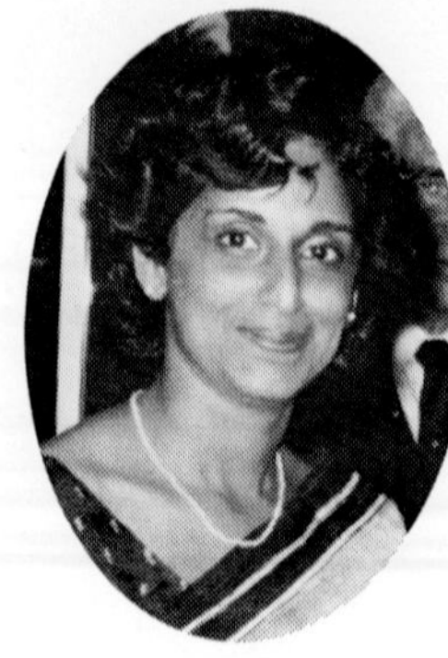

Dr. U. Surti

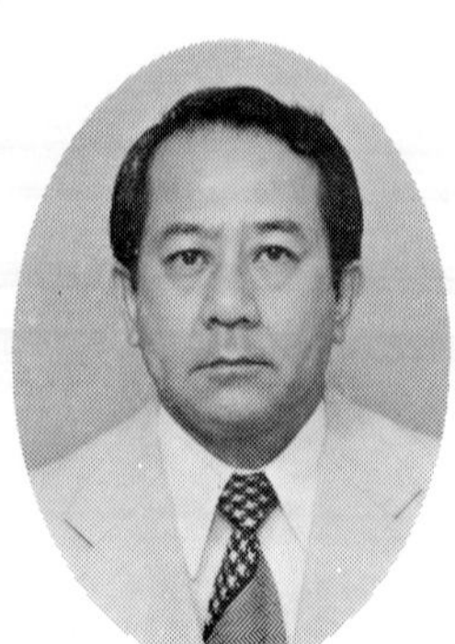

Dr. M. Mochizuki

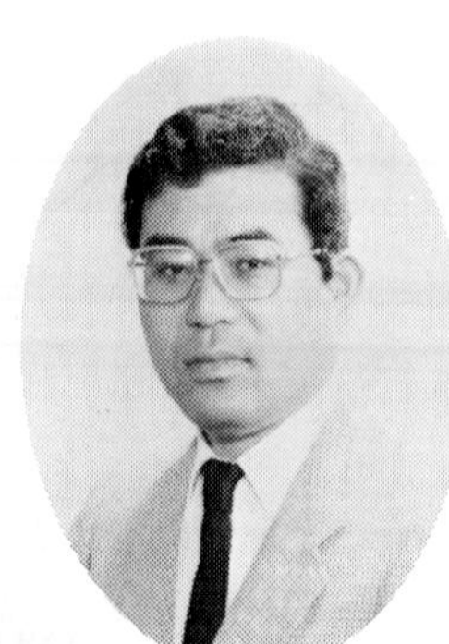

Dr. N. Wake

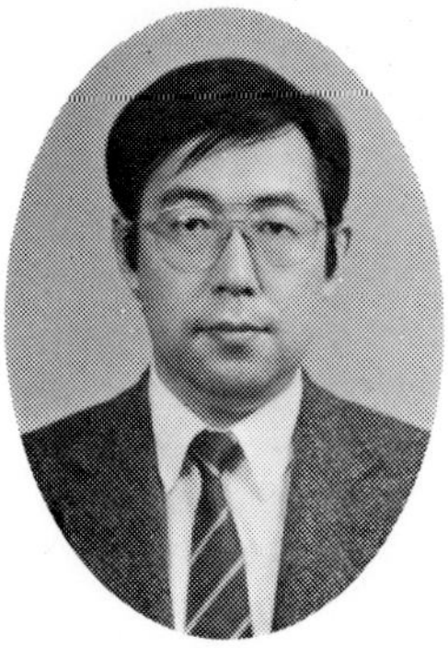
Dr. N. Sakuragi

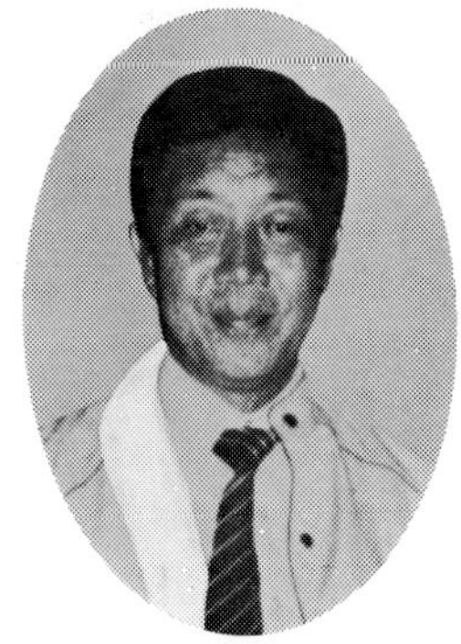
Dr. P. C. Wu

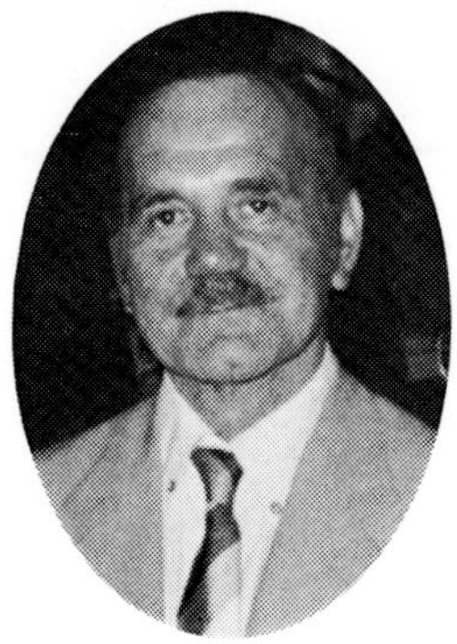
Dr. R. A. Pattillo

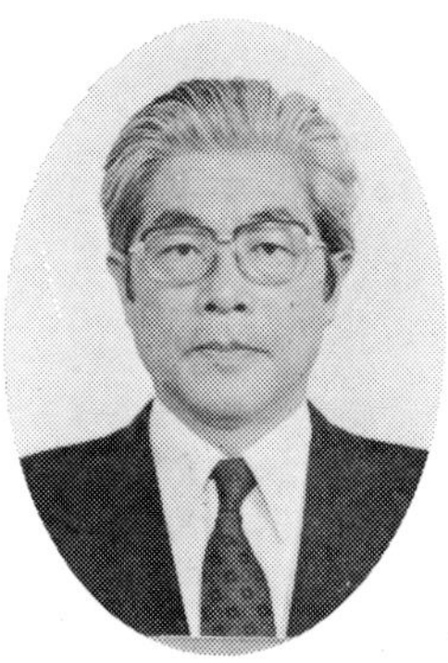
Dr. T. Fukushima

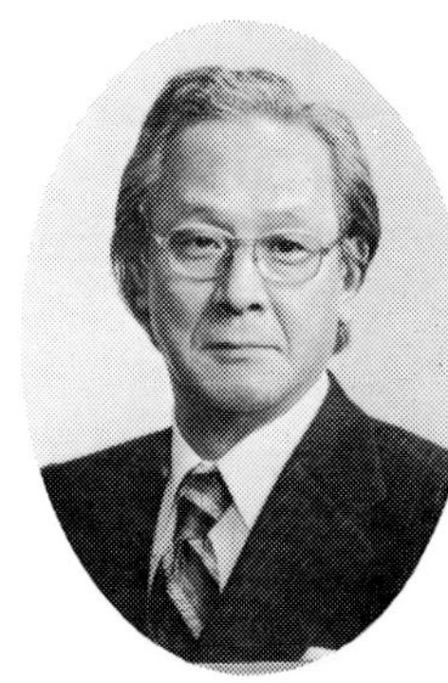
Dr. S. Takeuchi

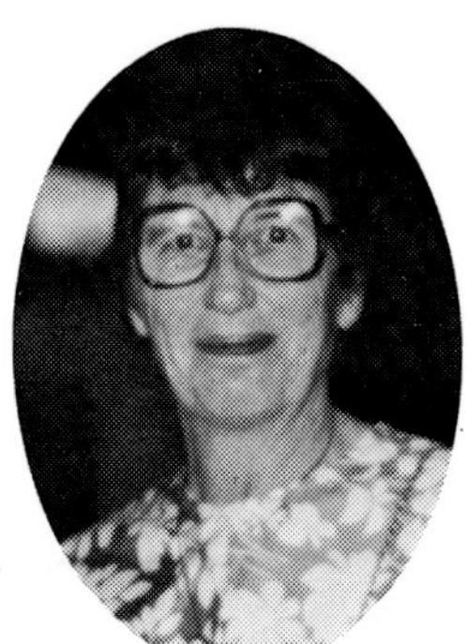
Dr. S. D. Lawler

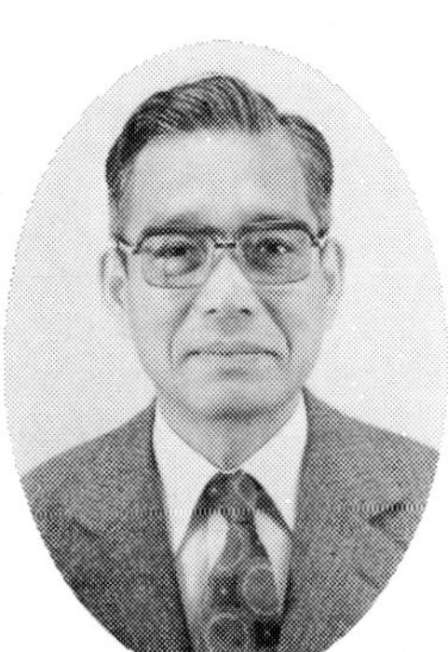
Dr. H. Takamizawa

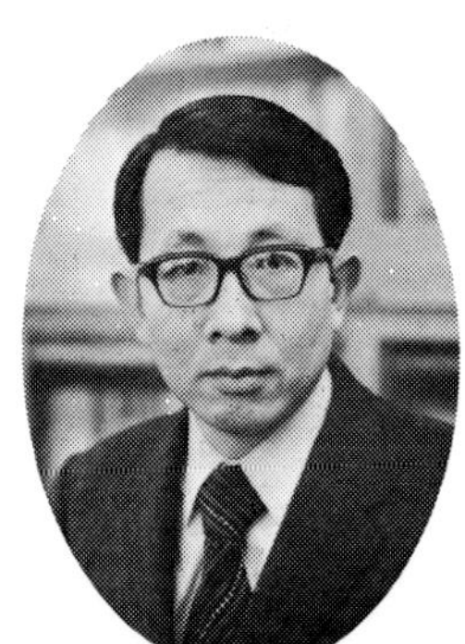
Dr. Y. Tomoda

Contributors

K.D. Bagshawe, M.D., F.R.C.P.
Department of Oncology, Cancer Research Campaign Laboratories, Charing Cross and Westminster Medical School, London W6 8RF, United Kingdom

R.H.J. Begent, M.D., M.R.C.P.
Department of Oncology, Cancer Research Campaign Laboratories, Charing Cross and Westminster Medical School, London W6 8RF, United Kingdom

Karin J. Blakemore, M.D.
Department of Obstetrics and Gynecology, Yale University School of Medicine, New Haven, CT 06510, U.S.A.

Darryl Carter, M.D.
Department of Obstetrics and Gynecology, Yale University School of Medicine, New Haven, CT 06510, U.S.A.

Joan Dent, R.N.
Department of Oncology, Cancer Research Campaign Laboratories, Charing Cross Hospital, London W6 8RF, United Kingdom

Rosemary A. Fisher, M.Phil.
Section of Genetics, Institute of Cancer Research and Royal Marsden Hospital, Fulham Road, London SW3 6JJ, United Kingdom

Tsutomu Fukuschima, M.D.
Department of Obstetrics and Gynecology, Sogo Kawasaki Chuo Hospital, 2-9-1 Tamachi, Kawasaki-ku, Kawasaki 210, Japan

Yoshihito Furuhashi, M.D.
Department of Obstetrics and Gynecology, School of Medicine, Nagoya University, Nagoya 466, Japan

Setsuko Gotoh, M.D.
Department of Obstetrics and Gynecology, School of Medicine, Nagoya University, Nagoya 466, Japan

Kazutaka Hamada, M.D.
Department of Obstetrics and Gynecology, Osaka City University School of Medicine, Osaka 545, Japan

Makoto Hoshina, M.D.
Department of Obstetrics and Gynecology, Kobe University School of Medicine, Kobe 650, Japan

Kihyoe Ichinoe, M.D.
Department of Obstetrics and Gynecology, Hokkaido University School of Medicine, Sapporo 060, Japan

Takao Ishizuka, M.D.
Department of Obstetrics and Gynecology, School of Medicine, Nagoya University, Nagoya 466, Japan

Barry M. Kacinski, M.D., Ph.D.
Department of Obstetrics and Gynecology, Yale University School of Medicine, New Haven, CT 06510, U.S.A.

Shigeaki Kaseki, M.D.
Department of Obstetrics and Gynecology, School of Medicine, Nagoya University, Nagoya 466, Japan

Sachihito Katoh, M.D.
Department of Obstetrics and Gynecology, School of Medicine, Nagoya University, Nagoya 466, Japan

Osamu Kobayashi, M.D.
Department of Obstetrics and Gynecology, Chiba University School of Medicine, Chiba 280, Japan

Ernest I. Kohorn, M.D.
Department of Obstetrics and Gynecology, Yale University School of Medicine, New Haven, CT 06510, U.S.A.

Sylvia D. Lawler, M.D.
Section of Genetics, Institute of Cancer Research and Royal Marsden Hospital, Fulham Road London SW3 6JJ, United Kingdom

Hisao Mano, M.D.
Department of Obstetrics and Gynecology, School of Medicine, Nagoya University, Nagoya 466, Japan

Takeshi Maruo, M.D.
Department of Obstetrics and Gynecology, Kobe University School of Medicine, Kobe 650, Japan

Hideo Matsui, M.D.
Department of Obstetrics and Gynecology, Chiba University School of Medicine, Chiba 280, Japan

Maria J. Merino, M.D.
Department of Obstetrics and Gynecology, Yale University School of Medicine, New Haven, CT 06510, U.S.A.

Matsuto Mochizuki, M.D.
Department of Obstetrics and Gynecology, Kobe University School of Medicine, Kobe 650, Japan

E.S. Newlands, Ph.D., F.R.C.P.
Department of Oncology, Cancer Research Campaign Laboratories, Charing Cross and Westminster Medical School, London W6 8RF, United Kingdom

Ryuichiro Nishimura, M.D.
Department of Obstetrics and Gynecology, Kobe University School of Medicine, Kobe 650, Japan

Kenichi Okudera, M.D.
Department of Obstetrics and Gynecology, Tokyo Medical College, Tokyo 160, Japan

Tatsuya Oosaki, M.D.
Department of Obstetrics and Gynecology, Chiba University School of Medicine, Chiba 280, Japan

Roland A. Pattillo, M.D.
Department of Obstetrics and Gynecology, Medical College of Wisconsin, Milwaukee, WI 53226, U.S.A.

G.J.S. Rustin, M.D., M.R.C.P.
Department of Oncology, Cancer Research Campaign Laboratories, Charing Cross and Westminster Medical School, London W6 8RF, United Kingdom

Noriaki Sakuragi, M.D.
Department of Obstetrics and Gynecology, Hokkaido University School of Medicine, Sapporo 060, Japan

Saumyendra Sarkar, Ph.D.
Department of Obstetrics and Gynecology, Yale University School of Medicine, New Haven, CT 06510, U.S.A.

Souei Sekiya, M.D.
Department of Obstetrics and Gynecology, Chiba University School of Medicine, Chiba 280, Japan

Hiroaki Soma, M.D.
Department of Obstetrics and Gynecology, Tokyo Medical College, Tokyo 160, Japan

Song Hong-Zhau, B.S., M.D.
Department of Obstetrics and Gynecology, Peking Union Medical College, Beijing, China

Tadashi Sugawa, M.D.
Department of Obstetrics and Gynecology, Osaka City University School of Medicine, Osaka 545, Japan

Urvashi Surti, Ph.D.
Department of Pathology, Magee-Womens Hospital, Pittsburgh, PA 15213, U.S.A.

A.E. Szulman, M.B.
Department of Pathology, Magee-Womens Hospital, Pittsburgh, PA 15213, U.S.A.

Hiroyoshi Takamizawa, M.D.
Department of Obstetrics and Gynecology, Chiba University School of Medicine, Chiba 280, Japan

Shoshichi Takeuchi, M.D.
Department of Obstetrics and Gynecology, Niigata University School of Medicine, Niigata 951, Japan
Toshitsugu Tamura, M.D.
Department of Obstetrics and Gynecology, Osaka City University School of Medicine, Osaka 545, Japan
Tang Min Yi, M.D.
Department of Obstetrics and Gynecology, Peking Union Medical College, Beijing, China
Yutaka Tomoda, M.D.
Department of Obstetrics and Gynecology, School of Medicine, Nagoya University, Nagoya 466, Japan
Naohiko Umesaki, M.D.
Department of Obstetrics and Gynecology, Osaka City University School of Medicine, Osaka 545, Japan
Wu Pao-Chen, B.S., M.D.
Department of Obstetrics and Gynecology, Peking Union Medical College, Beijing, China
Shizuko Yamabe, B.S.
Department of Obstetrics and Gynecology, Tokyo Medical College, Tokyo 160, Japan
Yang Xiu-Yu, B.S., M.D.
Department of Obstetrics and Gynecology, Peking Union Medical College, Beijing, China

Contents

PART ONE

GENETICS OF TROPHOBLASTIC DISEASES

1

Mechanisms of Origin of Hydatidiform Mole and Its Propensity to Malignancy

Kihyoe Ichinoe

Complete mole is an abnormal human pregnancy characterized by grossly swollen villi in the absence of a fetus. This often progresses in invasive moles or choriocarcinoma. The latter is a highly malignant tumor, though complete remission can be obtained despite widespread metastases. Not only is complete mole the major risk factor for choriocarcinoma (relative risk 2000–4000, possibly making it one of the largest single risk factors known for any disease), but the biological properties of both diseases are especially intriguing.

ANDROGENETIC ORIGIN OF COMPLETE MOLES

Complete moles show a distorted sex ratio. A vast majority of them have a 46,XX karyotype. This strange phenomenon was indicated for the first time from data resulting from the investigation of the incidence of sex chromatin-positive cells of complete moles (Table 1). The same had been also confirmed with the observation of Y-spot in molar cells. Figure 1, left side, shows the distribution of Y-spot-positive cells in trophoblasts of male and female conceptuses. Those results suggest that sex determination using quinacrine fluorescence was accurate. Thus the data shown on the right side suggest that Y-spot-negative cases are predominant in complete moles [3]. For similar purposes, the karyotype in 114 complete moles has been examined by Ichinoe [4]; 106 cases had an XX sex chromosome constitution, indicating that almost 93% of moles were genetically female (Table 2). The distorted sex ratio of the mole could not be explained by the idea that complete mole arose from normal fertilization. Thus, examinations using a variety of polymorphic features were performed to shed light on this strange phenomenon, and

Table 1. Frequency of positive sex chromatin in complete mole

Authors		Cases	Barr body (+)
Park	(1957)	22	16
Seer	(1958)	5	4
Harden	(1961)	22	19
Marquez	(1963)	50	38
Klinger et al.	(1966)	53	49
Tominaga et al.	(1966)	19	18
Beischer et al.	(1968)	137	101
Baggish et al.	(1968)	90	79
Westerhout et al.	(1969)	51	46
Total		449	369 (82%)

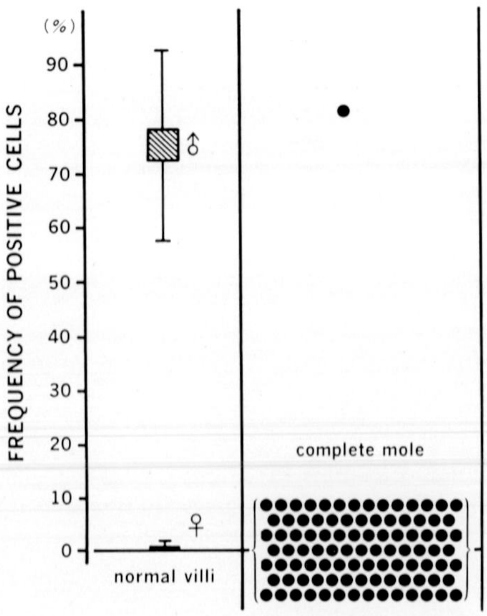

Figure 1. Distribution of Y-spot-positive cases in trophoblasts of normal conceptuses and complete moles. It was shown that Y-spot-negative cases were predominant in the latter.

Table 2. Sex chromosomal analysis of complete mole

No. of cases examined	XX	XY
114	106	8

presented interesting evidence that complete moles are androgenetic in origin [5, 7, 12, 13]. Six pairs of marker chromosomes of the representative mole and its parents are shown in Figure 2. Comparison of polymorphic markers indicates that neither of the maternal homologues was transmitted to the mole and both homologous chromosomes in the mole were traceable only to the one of corresponding paternal homologues. Investigations of human leukocyte antigen HLA (Table 3) and phosphoglucomutase-1 PGM_1 (Table 4) heteromorphisms between the mole and its parents also support the chromosomal data [6, 9, 17, 18], which suggest strongly that the mole received a paternal haploid set in duplicate, but none from the mother. This sequence leads to the preponderance of 46,XX karyotype in moles, as YY specimens are nonviable and lost during early

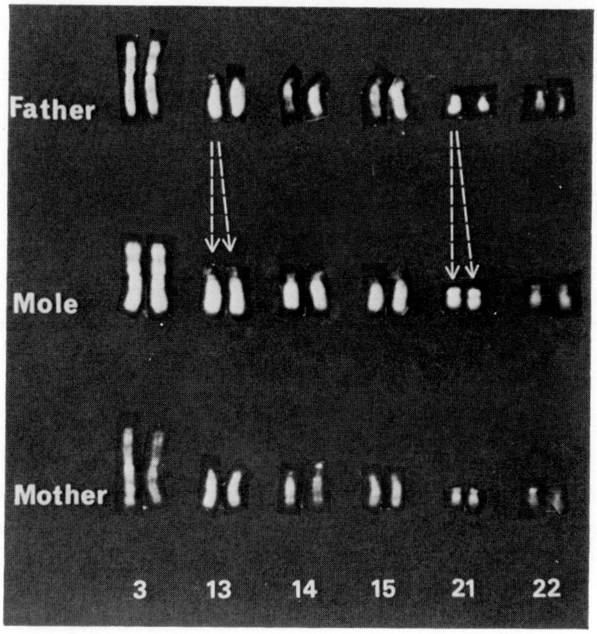

Figure 2. Six pairs of marker chromosomes of the representative mole and its parents. Comparison of polymorphic markers indicated that neither of the maternal homologues was transmitted to the mole and both homologous chromosomes in the mole were traceable only to the one of corresponding paternal homologues.

Table 3. HLA A- and B-types in complete moles and their parents

Case	Mole				Father				Mother			
	A locus		B locus		A locus		B locus		A locus		B locus	
1	A 2	—	B 5	—	A 2	Aw 9	B 5	Bw35	A 9	—	B 5	B 7
2	A 9	—	B 7	—	A 2	A 9	B 7	Bw54	A10	Aw19	Bw35	B40
3	A 9	—	B40	—	A 9	—	B40	Bw54	A 2	—	B15	—
4	A11	—	B40	—	A11	—	B 7	B40	A 2	A 9	B40	—
5	A 2	—	B 7	—	A 2	A10	B 7	—	A 2	A 9	B40	—
6	A11	—	Bw51	—	A 9	A11	Bw51	B 7	A 3	—	B13	Bw54
7	A 3	—	B40	—	A 3	A10	B40	Bw22	A 2	—	B40	Bw35
8	A 2	—	B 7	—	A 2	A 9	B 5	B 7	A10	—	B15	—
9	A 2	—	B40	—	A 2	A10	B40	—	A 2	—	B15	Bw22
10	A 9	—	Bw51	—	A 9	—	B 7	Bw51	A 9	A10	B 7	B40
11	A10	—	B40	—	A 2	A10	B40	—	A 2	A 9	B40	—
12	A 2	—	B40	—	A 2	Aw19	Bw13	B40	A 9	—	B 7	—
13	Aw24	—	B13	—	Aw24	—	Bw54	B13	A 2	A11	Bw51	Bw55
14	A26	—	Bw61	—	A 2	A26	Bw61	B13	Aw24	Aw33	Bw44	Bw62
15	A 2	—	Bw51	—	A 2	A26	Bw51	Bw35	A 2	Aw24	Bw51	Bw35
16	A26	—		—	A26	Aw24	Bw52	Bw62	Aw24	—	Bw61	—
17	Aw24	—	Bw52	—	Aw24	Aw33	Bw52	Bw44	A 2	Aw33	Bw44	Bw39
18	A 2	—	Bw55	—	A 2	A26	Bw55	Bw39	A 2	Aw33	Bw44	Bw38

stages of cleavage.

These observations indicate that "an empty egg" resulting from either enucleation or inactivation of the female pronucleus, is fertilized by either 1) a haploid sperm that is

Table 4. Parental origin of molar PGM_1 type in which the paternal type was heterozygous

Case	Mole	Father	Mother
1	1 — 1	1 — 2	1 — 1
2	1 — 1	1 — 2	1 — 2
3	1 — 1	1 — 2	1 — 2
4	1 — 1	1 — 2	1 — 2
5	1 — 1	1 — 2	1 — 2
6	2 — 2	1 — 2	1 — 1
7	1 — 1	1 — 2	1 — 2
8	1 — 1	1 — 2	1 — 1
9	2 — 2	1 — 2	1 — 1
10	1 — 1	1 — 2	1 — 1
11	1 — 1	1 — 2	2 — 2
12	1 — 1	1 — 2	2 — 2
13	1 — 1	1 — 2	1 — 1
14	1 — 1	1 — 2	1 — 1

duplicated without cytokinesis, or 2) a diploid sperm resulting from the failure of the second meiotic division. Studies using polymorphic traits with loci that are situated far from the centromeres, and thus subject to occasional meiotic crossing-over and recombination, were able to determine which of the two possibilities is likely. The complete homozygosity of HLA and PGM_1 heteromorphisms in moles, including cases in which the father was known to be heterozygous, support the theory of a haploid sperm origin for most of the XX moles.

In 1982, Wallace et al. [16] using restriction endonuclease in situ polymorphisms of mitochondrial DNA, verified that mitochondrial DNA of the mole is maternally derived, whereas molar nuclear chromosomes are exclusively paternal in origin. These findings indicate that moles arise from the fusion of one or two sperm nuclei with a mature but functionally anucleate ovum.

RISK FACTORS FOR MOLAR CONCEPTIONS

The finding of "androgenetic origin of complete moles" has cast an entirely new light on the etiology of complete mole, because formation of an abnormal egg (with an either eliminated or inactivated nucleus) plays a crucial role in the development of moles. Thus study of the risk factors associated with molar conception also offers the possibility for insight into the mechanism inducing an abnormal ovum in female meiosis. The following risk factors were examined in the present study: 1) maternal age; 2) HLA specificities among moles and their parents; 3) age of onset of menarche; 4) ABO blood groups; and 5) the kind of antecedent pregnancies followed by molar conceptions. Statistically significant results were obtained from the former two factors.

Maternal Senescence

The study was based on the complete regional records in Wakayama (in the southern part of Japan) and Sapporo (in the northern part of Japan). The geography and weather of the two cities are markedly different. The incidence of moles in all pregnancies was similar between both cities when the age of mother was 34 years or less; incidences of approximately 2.4% and 1.9% Wakayama and Sapporo, respectively, were noted (Figure 3). However, a significant increase in risk of complete mole among mothers delivering at ages between 40 and 44 years, with a further dominant increase beyond age 45 was shown

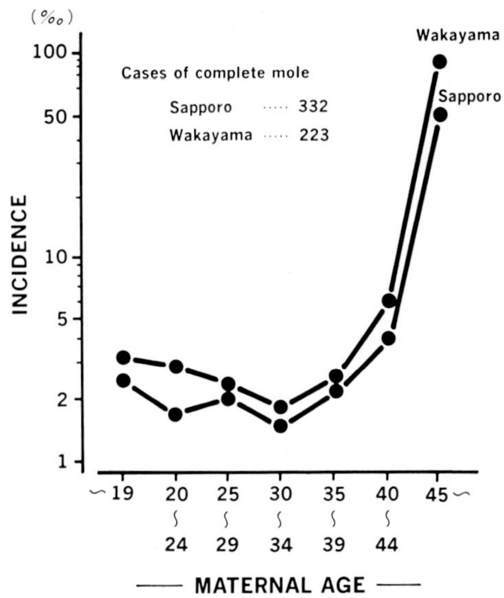

Figure 3. The incidence of molar conception and maternal age. The study was based on complete regional records in Wakayama and Sapporo, Japan, two cities in which the geography and weather are markedly different. A significant increase in risk of complete mole among mothers delivering after age 40 years was evident.

(Figure 3). These results suggest that the incidence of molar conception increases in parallel with the maternal senescence, especially beyond the age of 40 years. This seems to be the period when ovary malfunction and menopausal symptoms become evident in the female. It is generally well known that the incidence of pathologically abnormal ova increases in parallel with maternal senescence [11]. This thus suggests that maternal senescence plays an important role in the induction of a mature but functionally anucleate ovum. Data described elsewhere [2] showing increased nondisjunction frequency with senescence lead to the idea that expulsion of all chromosomes into the polar bodies is responsible for the formation of an empty egg. Somewhat less certain is whether or not very young women are also at an increased risk for complete moles.

HLA-A and -B Specificities among Moles and Their Parents

Complete mole is a form of natural allograft, as it carries only paternal genetic traits that differ antigenitically from those of the mother. Successful growth of mole is likely to be immunologically protected. Because the immune system is genetically controlled, the effect of the HLA system on the development of androgenetic ova into moles is of interest. Therefore, in the present study, HLA-A and -B specificities typed in the mole and its parent were compared with those of the general population in Japan. Results suggest that couples possessing some HLA types show excess risks for molar conception; groups composed of A2 fathers with A2 mothers, A2 fathers with A26 mothers or A26 fathers with A2 mothers had a statistically significant risk ($p<0.05$) (Table 5). However, the role of these two specificities for the development of moles remains unknown.

Table 6 shows HLA types observed in the complete mole. Again, the incidence of the A2 type was significantly higher than in the general population ($p<0.05$). The high incidence of the A2 type in moles would reflect the androgenetic origin because it was also significantly high in fathers; most moles inherit the paternal genome in duplicate.

Table 5. Maternal age dependence of chromosome aberrations in induced abortions (before 12 weeks' pregnancy)

Age group	Chromosome analysis			
	No. of cases	Abnormalities	Karyotype	(Trisomy %)
35–39	231	21 (9.5%)	Trisomy: G (6), D (5), E (4), A (1), B (1), C (1)	18 (8.1%)
			XO (1)	
			Trans. (1)	
			Triploidy (1)	
40–44	299	51 (17.1%)	Trisomy: G (13), D (6), E (7), A (2), B (2), C (8), F (2)	40 (13.4%)
			Double trisomy (2)	
			XO (2)	
			Trans. (1)	
			Triploidy (4)	
			Mosaicism (2)	
45–48	24	8 (33.3%)	Trisomy: G (3), D (1), E (3)	7 (29.2%)
			Double trisomy (1)	
Total	544	80 (14.7%)		65 (11.9%)

Table 6. Gene frequencies of parents with molar conception

Father — Mother	Gene frequency in Japanese population			
	Molar development		Normal development	
A 2 —— A 2	7.0%	>	3.5%	(p<0.05)
A 2 —— A26	3.1%	>	1.4%	(p<0.05)
A26 —— A 2	3.0%	>	1.4%	(p<0.05)
Other combinations	....			No significance

Table 7. Gene frequencies of HLA types in complete moles and their parents

HLA types	Father (n=87)	Mother (n=96)	Mole (n=52)	General population in Japan (n=495)
A–2	29.70*	23.62	41.17*	18.81*
–9	5.31	6.46	13.40	27.96
–11	7.15	10.44	11.21	8.92
–24	27.29	23.02	25.32	27.45
–26	12.90	10.44	3.92	7.49
B–35	7.77	9.86	3.92	7.23
–44	4.71	7.58	1.94	9.99
–54	5.92	5.90	0.00	7.12
Bw–61	6.54	7.02	6.97	9.66
–62	7.15	8.14	2.93	6.69

* (p<0.05)

Table 8. Compatibility of HLA A- and B-types among parents and their moles

A. Compatible						26 cases	26/30 (86.7%)
—Representative cases—							
1) For two types						4 cases	
	Father	A 2	Aw26	Bw51	Bw35		
	Mother	A 2	Aw24	Bw51	Bw35		
	Mole	A 2		Bw51			
2) For one type						22 cases	
	Father	A 2	A10	B 7			
	Mother	A 2	A 9	Bw22	B40		
	Mole	A 2		B 7			
	Father	A26	—	Bw52	—		
	Mother	A 2	Aw31	Bw52	B27		
	Mole	A24	—	Bw52	—		
B. Incompatible						4 cases	4/30 (13.3%)
—Representative cases—							
	Father	Aw24	Aw31	Bw52	Bw62		
	Mother	Aw24	Aw33	Bw52	Bw44		
	Mole		Aw31		Bw62		

The incidence of couples, and of the mole and the mother possessing at least one identical A or B specificity, was 59.8% and 50.0%, respectively (Tables 7 and 8). Because the compatibility ratio of the random population was 60.5% [8], there was no statistically significant difference. However, the ratio in which the HLA type identical to both parents was inherited into the mole, was 86.7% (Table 9). This was significantly higher than the value estimated from the type of inheritance in androgenetic moles (67.3%). This suggests that compatibility of HLA system among moles and their parents may be important for the growth and the cell proliferation of androgenetic conceptuses, though their haplotype remains to be clarified.

RISK FACTORS FOR POSTMOLAR TROPHOBLASTIC DISEASES

Complete mole has a propensity toward residual trophoblastic disease, invasive mole, and choriocarcinoma. It has been widely accepted in Japan that 10% to 20% of moles develop postmolar trophoblastic diseases. However, the exact mechanisms that promote the progression of moles into trophoblastic diseases are not well elaborated. Thus a variety of risk factors representing characteristics of molar trophoblasts and status of hosts were evaluated. Significant results were obtained from investigations for the zygosity of molar cells and for the maternal aging.

Zygosity of Molar Cells

There are two main mechanisms of origin for complete mole. More than 90% of moles result from fertilization of an empty egg by a haploid sperm. The paternally derived haploid set then duplicates without cytokinesis and restores diploidy. Invariably, this class of moles has a 46,XX karyotype and is completely homozygous for any genetic markers. Fertilization of an empty egg by two spermatozoa is responsible for the remaining cases [10].

The androgenetic origin of complete mole has provided us with a means for directly evaluating the relationship between choriocarcinomas and their putative forerunners;

Table 9. Parental origin of genetic markers in heterozygous moles

Case		Karyotype (Y-body)	Chromosome 3	4	13	14	15	21	22	HLA A-locus		B-locus		PGM_1
	Father									A 9,	A10	Bw51,	Bw16	
1	Mole									A 9,	A10	Bw51,	Bw16	
	Mother									A 2,	A 9	Bw51,	—	
	Father		ab	aa	ab	ab	ab	aa	ab	A 2,	—	Bw51,	Bw55	2—1
2	Mole	46,XY	ab	aa	ab	aa	aa	aa	ab	A 2,	—	Bw51,	Bw55	2—1
	Mother		aa	aa	cc	aa	cd	aa	cc	A11,	Aw24	B 7,	Bw60	1—1
	Father									A 2,	A26	Bw51,	—	1—1
3	Mole	Y-body (+)								A26,	—	Bw51,	—	1—1
	Mother									A26,	Aw31	Bw44,	Bw62	2—2
	Father													
4	Mole	46,XY	aa	aa	aa	ab	aa	aa	aa					2—2
	Mother		ab	aa	bb	aa	bb	bb	bc					1—1
	Father		ab	ab	ab	aa	ab	ab	ab	A 2,	A11	Bw52,	Bw35	2—1
5	Mole	46,XX	aa	ab	bb	aa	aa	ab	ab	A 2,	A11	Bw52,	Bw35	1—1
	Mother		ab	bc	bb	aa	ab	bb	ab	Aw24,	—	B37 ,	—	2—2
	Father									A 2,	Aw24	Bw60,	Bw46	1—2
6	Mole									A 2,	Aw24	Bw60,	Bw46	2—2
	Mother									A11,	A26	Bw48,	Bw62	1—1
	Father									A 2,	—	B 7 ,	Bw39	
7	Mole	46,XX	aa	aa	aa	aa	aa	aa	ab	A 2,	—	B 7 ,	Bw39	
	Mother									A 2,	A26	Bw60,	Bw62	
	Father									A 2,	A11	Bw61,	Bw59	
8	Mole									A 2,	—	Bw61,	Bw59	
	Mother									A 2,	—	Bw54,	Bw62	
	Father													
9	Mole	Y-body (+)												
	Mother													
	Father													
10	Mole	Y-body (+)												
	Mother													

complete homozygosity and/or exclusive inheritance of a paternal genome would be expected if the tumor arose from complete mole. A study of five cases of choriocarcinoma showed overt heterozygosity (Figure 4) [14, 15]. Apparently, these tumors did not originate from complete moles of monospermic origin. If the association between complete mole and choriocarcinoma is true, it may be assumed that dispermic moles are more prone to malignancy than are monospermic, homozygous moles.

The validity of this assumption was tested by performing follow-up studies of patients after evacuation of mono- and dispermic moles. Follow-up of patients consisted mainly of the measurement of urinary human chorionic gonadotropin (hCG). In the present study, cases in which the urinary hCG was higher than 1,000 IU/liter at the 5th week, 100 IU/liter at the 8th week, and/or the luteinizing hormone (LH) level was not obtained at the 12th week by the urinary hCG examination after evacuation of moles were considered to have postmolar trophoblastic disease.

Chromosomal, HLA, and PGM_1 polymorphisms were studied to explore zygosity in 61 complete moles. Of these, 51 were homozygous for every tested marker. These cases,

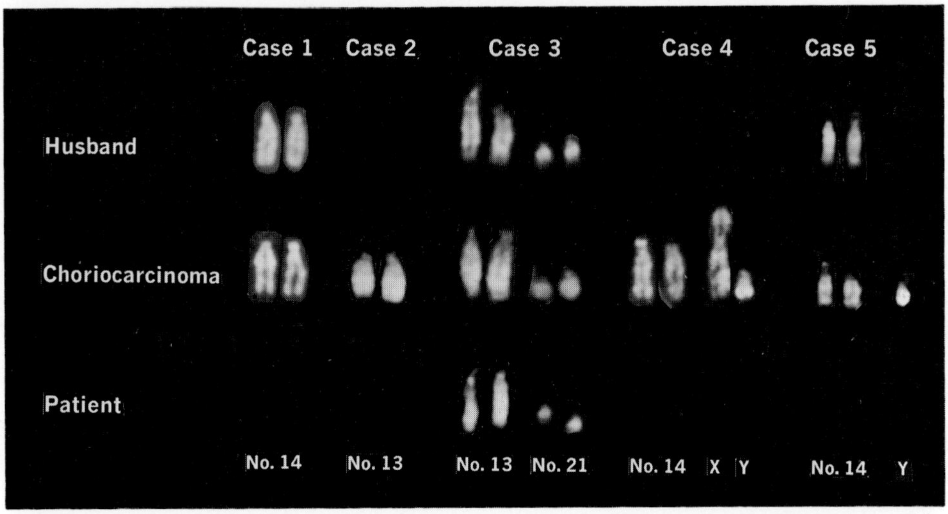

Figure 4. Overt heterozygosity is shown in five cases of choriocarcinoma. Heterozygosity could be confirmed with the comparison of polymorphic features of marker chromosomes and the sex chromosome constitution.

Table 10. Incidence of postmolar trophoblastic diseases in homozygous and heterozygous moles

	No. of cases examined	No. of cases with postmolar trophoblastic diseases	Unclassified	Invasive mole	Choriocarcinoma
Androgenic moles	85	16 (17.9%)	11	4	1
Homozygous	51	7 (13.7%)	6	1	0
Heterozygous	10	5 (50.0%)	3	2	0
Unknown zygosity	24	4 (16.7%)	2	1	1

Table 11. Incidence of lung metastases in complete moles

Moles	No. of cases examined	No. of cases	
		Postmolar trophoblastic disease	Lung metastases
Homozygous	51	7 (13.7%)	0
Heterozygous	10	5 (50.0%)	2 (20.0%)

having a 46,XX karyotype, were most probably derived from an empty egg fertilized by a 23,X spermatozoon. Ten moles were heterozygous for at least one genetic marker. Most probably, these moles were the products of an empty egg fertilized by two spermatozoa (Table 10).

Of 61 cases, 12 (19.8%) required chemotherapy due to the reelevation or the high level of urinary hCG (Table 11). Of 51 homozygous moles, 7 showed a plateauing high hCG titer. Incidence of postmolar trophoblastic diseases was 13.7%. However, malignant sequelae occurred in five of ten patients who had had heterozygous moles. The incidence was 50.0% and was higher than that of homozygous moles, although the number of cases examined was too small for statistical analysis.

The clinical course of seven patients with postmolar trophoblastic diseases after evacuation of homozygous moles are shown in Figure 5. There was no case with lung metastases. Most cases were suspected to have residual but degenerating trophoblasts in the uterine

Homozygous moles

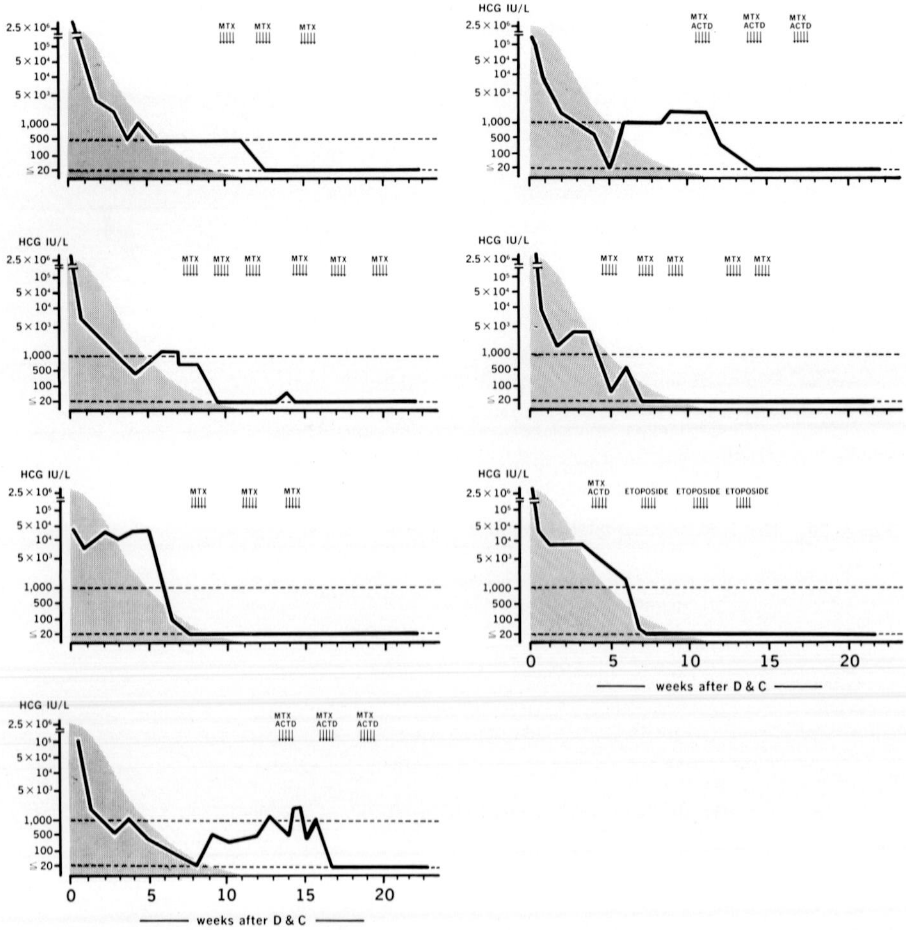

Figure 5. Clinical courses of seven patients with postmolar trophoblastic diseases after evacuation of homozygous 46,XX moles. There was no case with lung metastases, and most cases were suspected to have residual but degenerating trophoblasts in the uterine cavity in view of the relatively low urinary hCG levels and quick response to chemotherapy.

cavity in view of the relatively low urinary hCG levels and quick response to chemotherapy. The clinical course of five patients with postmolar trophoblastic diseases after evacuation of heterozygous moles are shown in Figure 6. The hCG levels of these cases were absolutely higher than in the cases of homozygous mole, and two of five cases had multiple lung metastases. A severe degree of complications with high hCG titer and metastases was assumed to have developed from heterozygous moles. This leads to the hypothesis that the homozygous mole is a strong proliferative disadvantage, possibly because of homozygosity for recessive mutations at certain loci necessary for autonomous cell proliferation. These trophoblasts would disappear before malignant transformation. This hypothesis may also explain the failure of some heterozygous moles to become malignant because of chance homozygosity for the same putative recessive mutations, as well as

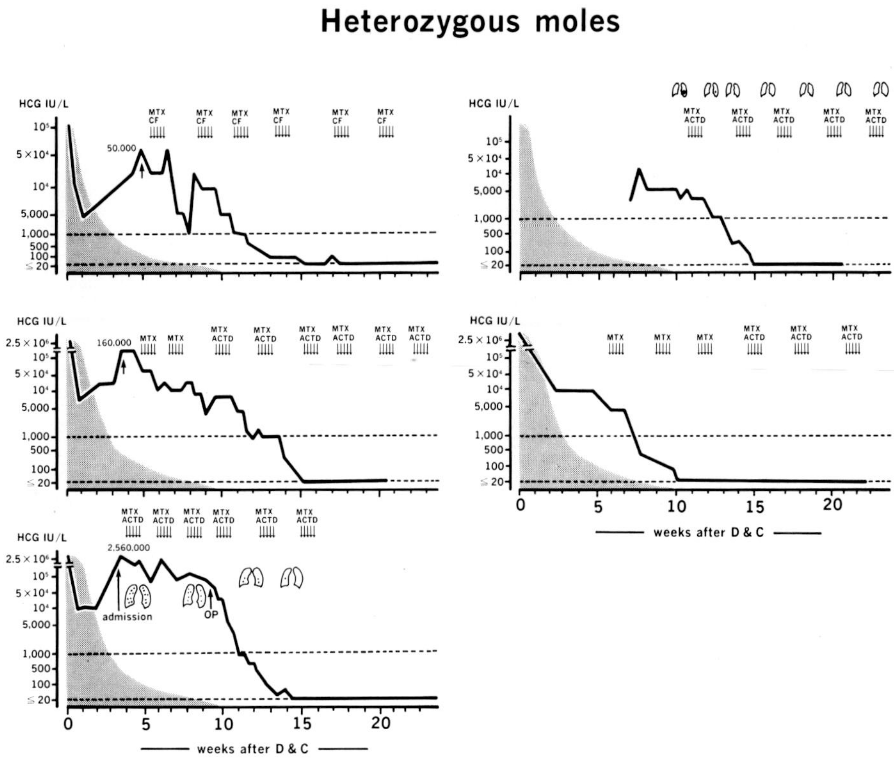

Figure 6. Clinical courses of five patients with postmolar trophoblastic diseases after evacuation of heterozygous moles. The hCG levels of these cases were higher than those with homozygous moles, and two of the five cases had multiple lung metastases.

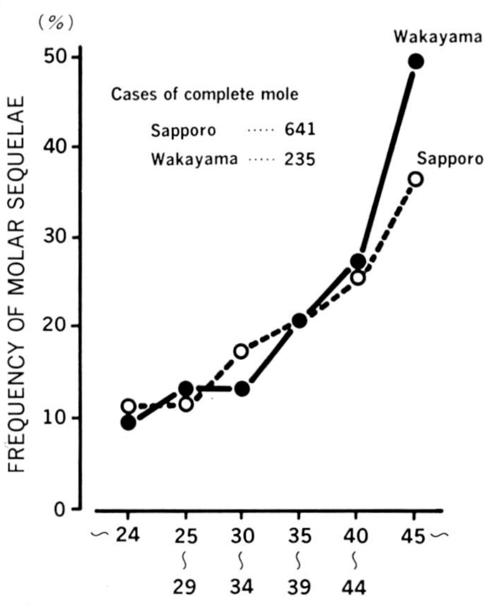

Figure 7. The increased incidence of postmolar trophoblastic diseases in older women. The incidence of postmolar trophoblastic diseases rose from 12.7% in women under the age of 34 years to 27.2% in those over the age of 35 years.

the rare homozygous moles that undergo malignant transformation because they lack such lethal mutations. As a result, it was assumed that the heterozygosity observed in molar cells was one of major risk factors for postmolar trophoblastic diseases.

Maternal Aging

Maternal factors that promote the progression of moles to trophoblastic diseases are not well elaborated, although several studies have shown higher risks of progression for mothers who develop a complete mole at an older age [1]. Also, in the present study the incidence of postmolar trophoblastic diseases rose from 12.7% in women under the age of 34 years to 27.2% in those over the age of 35 years, with high significance (Figure 7). In particular, an extraordinarily enlarged incidence at the age of over 45 years is noted. It is also evident that the incidence of postmolar choriocarcinoma increases with maternal age, especially in women over the age of 40 years (Figure 8). However, the zygosity of molar trophoblasts needs to be accounted for in the interpretation of these statistics. Thus, the age distribution of patients with Y-spot-positive and dispermic moles has been investigated. An increase of those moles in patients over the age of 40 years is perhaps possible (Table 12), though the number of cases was relatively small. This suggests that maternal aging is also a risk factor for malignant complications even if the association between the incidence of dispermic moles and, maternal senescence has been suggested. Overall frequencies of 1) the HLA-A and -B locus antigens, 2) ABO blood groups, 3) age of onset of menarche, 4) duration of molar conceptions and 5) urinary hCG level before the evacua-

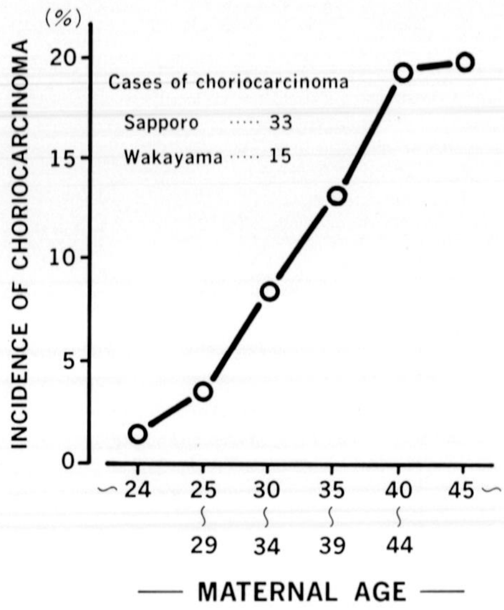

Figure 8. The incidence of postmolar choriocarcinoma and materral age. The enlarged incidence of choriocarcinoma in women over the age of 40 years is shown.

Table 12. Maternal age and incidence of dispermic complete moles and Y-spot-positive moles

Age	No. of cases	Karyotype	%	No. of cases	Y-spot (+)	%
–19	3	1		9	1	11.1
20–29	31	5	16.1	65	4	6.1
30–39	14	3	17.1	23	0	0
40–49	6	1	16.7	12	2	16.2
Total	54	10	18.5	109	7	6.4

tion among moles developing trophoblastic diseases and their parents have not differed significantly from those observed in cases without sequelae.

As a result, two risk factors for molar conceptions and two risk factors that promote progression to trophoblastic diseases could be evaluated in the present study. Regarding the former, it was assumed that maternal age plays an important role for the induction of a mature but functionally anucleated ovum, and compatibility of HLA systems among moles and their parents is important for the growth and the cell proliferation of androgenetic conceptuses.

Zygosity of molar cells and maternal age could be evaluated as "risk factors for postmolar trophoblastic diseases". The former may represent the vigor of molar trophoblasts and the latter may be affected by environmental and biological factors of the host. However, these are not directly responsible for choriocarcinogenesis. Therefore, it is absolutely necessary to explore the transformation mechanisms of molar trophoblasts in the near future.

REFERENCES

1. Bracken MB, Brinton LA, Hayashi K: Epidemiology of hydatidiform mole and choriocarcinoma. Epidemiol Rev 6: 52–75, 1984.
2. Fujimoto S, Tsuji K, Ichinoe K: Maternal age dependence of chromosome aberrations in induced abortions. Proc Jpn Acad 54: 601–606, 1978.
3. Ichinoe K, Shiina Y, Wake N, Hoshi S: Cytogenetic studies on molar genesis. Asia Oceania J Obstet Gynecol 7: 123–134, 1981.
4. Ichinoe K: Unpublished data.
5. Jacobs PA, Hassold TJ, Matsuyama AM, Newlands IM: Chromosome constitution of gestational trophoblastic disease. Lancet 2: 49, 1978.
6. Jacobs PA, Wilson CM, Sprenkle JA, Rosenshein NB, Migeon BR: Mechanism of origin of complete hydatidiform moles. Nature 286: 714–716, 1980.
7. Kajii T, Ohama K: Androgenetic origin of hydatidiform mole. Nature 268: 633–634, 1977.
8. Kuroda M: Unpublished data.
9. Lawler SD, Pickthall VJ, Fisher RA, Povey S, Evans MW, Szulman AE: Genetic studies of complete and partial hydatidiform moles. Lancet 2: 580, 1979.
10. Ohama K, Kajii T, Ikamoto E, Fukuda Y, Imaizumi K, Tsukahara M, Kobayashi K, Hagiwara K: Dispermic origin of XY hydatidiform moles. Nature 292: 551–552, 1981.
11. Okada Y, Ichinoe K: The occurrence rate of neonatal anomaly related to aging of grafted ovaries in mice. Acta Obstet Gynecol Jpn 33: 222–228, 1981.
12. Wake N, Shiina Y, Ichinoe K: A further cytogenetic study of hydatidiform mole, with reference to its androgenetic origin. Proc Jpn Acad 54: 533–537, 1978.
13. Wake N, Takagi N, Sasaki M: Androgenesis as a cause of hydatidiform mole. J Natl Cancer Inst 60: 51–57, 1978.
14. Wake N, Tanaka K, Chapman V, Matsui S, Sandberg AA: Chromosomes and cellular origin of choriocarcinoma. Cancer Res 41: 3137–3143, 1981.
15. Wake N, Ichinoe K: Unpublished data.
16. Wallace DC, Surti U, Adams CW, Szulman AE: Complete moles have paternal chromosomes but maternal mitochondrial DNA. Hum Genet 61: 145–147, 1982.
17. Yamashita K, Wake N, Araki T, Ichinoe K, Kuroda M: Human lymphocyte antigen expression in hydatidiform mole: Androgenesis following fertilization by a haploid sperm. Am J Obstet Gynecol 135: 597–600, 1979.
18. Yamashita K, Wake N, Araki T, Ichinoe K, Kuroda M: A further HLA study of hydatidiform moles. Gynecol Oncol 11: 23–28, 1981.

2

Genetics of Hydatidiform Moles: Pittsburgh Study

Urvashi Surti and A. E. Szulman

INTRODUCTION

Hydatidiform moles have been separated into two separate syndromes. Complete hydatidiform mole is a conceptus without a fetus with generalized swelling of all the villi with trophoblastic hyperplasia [20]. Microscopically one finds central cistern formation and random necrobiosis of the villus mesenchyme. The embryo dies early in development before the establishment of the fetal circulation, and fetal red blood cells are absent from the villous vessels. Complete moles have a diploid 46,XX or 46,XY karyotype of paternal origin.

With partial hydatidiform mole, the conceptus represents a dilute version of complete mole. A mixture of swollen and normal-appearing villi is found. Existence of a fetus can be ascertained by the presence of fetal red blood cells. Trophoblastic hyperplasia is inconspicuous but present. Scalloping of the villi and trophoblastic inclusions are the features that are present in partial moles, but absent in complete moles. Partial moles usually have a triploid karyotype with an additional set of chromosomes derived from the father. The detailed histological features are fully described elsewhere [24–28, 34].

The results of the genetic studies done on the moles received at Magee-Womens Hospital are briefly described in this communication. For a historical review the reader is referred to the recent article by Lawler [15].

In addition to routine cytogenetic analysis, the parental origin of both types of moles was determined by using chromosomal heteromorphisms, isozyme polymorphisms, and DNA restriction fragment length polymorphisms.

Cytogenetic Markers

The heritable difference between the chromosomes such as satellites and secondary constrictions have long been known [2]. With the advent Q- and C-banding, a wide range of chromosome polymorphisms can be recognized and used to study the origin of complete moles [11–13, 16, 18, 21, 22, 30]. Such markers on chromosomes 1, 3, 4, 9, 13, 14, 15, 16, 21, and 22 have made possible the determination of parental origin of the extra haploid set in many triploids [10, 14, 17]. Other techniques used for the same purpose are the analysis of blood group antigens [6] and of human leukocyte antigen (HLA) markers [4, 33]. From the data available at present, it seems that the extra set in triploidy is nearly always of paternal origin and mainly results from dispermy [8, 17].

Enzyme Studies: 46,XX Classical Moles

As the quinacrine markers are located on or very near the centromere, crossing-over in these regions should be minimal. The method does not distinguish between the two possible mechanisms by which the 46,XX moles could originate. In the first mechanism, there is duplication of a paternal single X-carrying haploid set (23,X), giving rise to a 46,XX mole. In this case one would expect 100% homozygosity at all the gene loci. So far, all of the 46,XX complete moles fall in this category [13, 17, 23, 24, 29]. In the second mechanism by which 46,XX moles could originate, a diploid sperm (46,XX) resulting from a failure of second meiotic division is responsible for the mole. In this case one would expect occasional heterozygosity in the mole as result of crossing-over during meiosis I.

Analysis of gene products of the loci away from the centromere would distinguish between the two possible mechanisms and would give additional clues as to the paternal or maternal origin of the molar genome.

We have been studying the moles and the parents for a series of polymorphic enzyme systems for this purpose. So far, we have analyzed for the following:

Enzyme	Location on human chromosome
1. PGM 1 (phosphoglucomutase-1)	1
2. PGD 6 (phosphogluconate dehydrogenase)	1
3. PGM3 (phosphoglucomutase-3)	6
4. GLO (glyoxalase)	6
5. ESD (esterase D)	13
6. PEPD (peptidase D)	19
7. ADA (adenosine deaminase)	20
8. G6PD (glucose 6 phosphate dehydrogenase)	X
9. AK (adenylate kinase)	9

To detect crossing-over, heterozygous loci in the fathers can be compared with the same loci in the respective moles. In case of a duplication of a single haploid sperm, the above-mentioned loci will be homozygous in the moles when the father is heterozygous. In case of the failure of second meiotic division, some of the loci in the moles will be heterozygous.

Enzyme analysis has been informative in elucidating and confirming the exact origin of both 46,XX and 46,XY complete moles [7, 16, 18, 21]. Enzyme analysis in triploid partial moles has not been as informative because enzyme levels can not easily be quantitated in terms of a single or double dose. Cytogenetic and restriction fragment length polymorphism (RFLP) analysis is much more successful in elucidating the origins of various moles than the enzyme analysis. In about 20% of cases origin can be inferred on the basis of enzymes alone in our series. In other cases enzyme data are used to confirm the results obtained by cytogenetics and RFLP.

Analysis of Restriction Fragment Length Polymorphisms

Most of the traditional genetic markers available (except HLA) are not sufficiently polymorphic to be informative in determination of the exact mechanism of origin in many cases of hydatidiform moles. A minimum degree of polymorphism in human DNA is calculated to be 1 in 1000 base pairs [3, 32]. Therefore new polymorphisms can be recognized by means of the restriction enzymes. These are site-specific endonucleases that recognize six or four base sequences at which the DNA is cut. The resultant fragments can be displayed according to their length by electrophoresis on agarose gel. Hybridization by Southern blotting technique using radioactive probes of single-copy DNA fragments can reveal a loss or gain of a restriction site in DNA of different individuals. Differences among individuals in the restriction fragment lengths are caused by individual base differences and result in a loss or gain of a restriction site, or insertion or deletion of blocks of DNA altering the size of the fragment. These polymorphisms have been successfully used in diagnosis of sickle cell disease, and in recognizing the maternal inheritance of mitochondrial DNA in humans. We have already used this tool to determine the origin of the mitochondrial DNA in complete moles, wherein the nuclear DNA is paternal and cytoplasmic DNA is of maternal origin [29]. In addition, substantial DNA amplification of any of the sequences tested can be identified. White and Leppert at the University of Utah have recognized a number of such polymorphisms and have collaborated in analyzing RFLP in our mole families. Probes currently in use include: Hras-1, the insulin gene (PINS 310), D11S12, a cloned sequence that reveals polymorphisms with MspI and BclI (chromosome 11). The arbitrary highly polymorphic probe D14S1 is found on chromosome 14. Probe DXY1 has homology to a 14 kb fragment on Y chromosome and reveals a polymorphism on X chromosome. Gamma globin gene hybridizing with gamma G and gamma A loci (chromosome 11) and beta globin gene probe (chromosome 16) are also used. The results of the cytogenetic and RFLP data where comparable are in complete agreement (Leppert et al., unpublished data). Whereas 16 complete moles are androgenic in origin and homozygous at every locus, 12 partial moles have a single maternal haploid set and two paternal haploid sets.

Although data on karyotypes were unavailable for five complete mole examples, the DNA probe DXYS1 uncovered no Y chromosome DNA sequences when hybridized to molar DNA. The data indicate that they are likely to be homozygous 46,XX. No obvious amplification was noticed for any of genes examined including H-Ras oncogene in diploid and triploid moles.

Several authenticated dispermic XY moles are on record, but no dispermic XX moles have been recorded. It would seem probable that 46,XX heterozygous moles may be missed and a multimethod search including RFLP is warranted.

RESULTS

We have 43 complete moles with exclusive paternal origin determined by heteromorphisms of chromosomes, isozymes, and RFLPs (unpublished data). Thirty-six cases are 46,XX and homozygous, whereas five cases have a 46,XY karyotype resulting from dispermy. Both parental bloods were available in 39 cases, and in nine cases only maternal blood was available. One recently seen complete mole has a triploid karyotype totally of paternal origin. One twin pregnancy was found to have one complete mole 46,XX of paternal origin and one normal fetus with normal paternal and maternal haploid set. All the above moles have the morphology of the complete syndrome.

It has been suggested that dispermic complete moles (46,XX and 46,XY) are more prone to persistent trophoblastic disease as opposed to homozygous 46,XX complete moles [5, 13, 15, 31]. A retrospective sex chaomatin (X and Y) analysis on moles with known and unknown karyotype and homozygous vs. heterozygous constitution performed in this laboratory showed slight increase in persistent trophoblastic disease after 46,XY moles [19]. The number of cases in our series as well as in the literature is too small for an unequivocal conclusion and further analysis of new cases is necessary [5, 12, 13, 30, 31].

Morphological and clinical data from a retrospective and prospective studies, including pre- and postoperative human chorionic gonadotropin (hCG) levels, have been analyzed at Magee-Womens Hospital from 1972 to 1984 (unpublished data). This series included 194 benign complete moles and 23 complete moles with residual trophoblast disease including choriocarcinomas. It contained also 295 partial moles with four cases of residual trophoblastic disease requiring chemotherapy; there were no cases of choriocarcinoma. Tissue culture and genetic studies were performed only on those cases that were obtained prospectively, as discussed above.

We had 119 cases of partial moles that came to the laboratory for culture in the last five years. Of these, 54 were found to be 69,XXY; 38 were 69,XXX; one was 69,XYY. There were 16 cases that failed to grow, 7 that were triploid, but had insufficient growth for complete analysis, two cases of partial moles that were 92,XXXY with a triple paternal contribution; and a single maternal contribution [23]. It seems that the formation of the mole is associated with an excess of the paternal over the maternal haploid contributions. This is supported by a recently proposed hypothesis that the maternal and paternal genomic contributions are not equivalent functionally, and that they undergo a separate specific imprinting during oogenesis and spermatogenesis, respectively [1]. Activiated enucleated murine eggs were reconstituted with exogenous male and female pronuclei. Only male plus female diploid combinations of pronuclei could give rise to normal embryos. Digynic diploids could not develop beyond a certain early postimplantation stage and produced a poor trophoblast even if the embryo proper developed to some degree. In contrast, reconstituted diandric eggs showed markedly better trophoblastic development, whereas the embryo itself died early. Such findings point to some dependence of the extraembryonic tissues, notably the trophoblast, on the paternal genome, whereas some maternal genes seem necessary for the development of the embryo proper.

In 69 partial moles there were two paternal sets and one maternal haploid set. In 14 cases digyny could not be ruled out, but all 14 were compatible with diandry. No case of unequivocal digynic partial mole was found. Enzyme and RFLP data were compatible with the above results.

One to two percent of all conceptions are triploid. The majority of cases are aborted in first or second trimester, and the few born alive die in first few days of life. It is now recognized that 85% of triploids have a placenta that is partially molar, 15% of triploids have a normal placenta, and there are no intermediate forms [26]. Jacobs and others (1978, 1982) have shown that the extra haploid set of chromosomes is of paternal origin in about 73% of triploids and of maternal origin in 27% of triploids [8, 9]. Correlation of the origin of the extra set of chromosomes and the morphology of the placenta in 107 triploids suggested that the development of partial mole is primarily associated with the presence of two paternal haploid sets, as all 57 diandric cases turned out to be partial moles and only 3 of 21 cases with two maternal sets were partial moles [9]. We believe that the case for the diandry partial mole association is still valid. This finding is in agreement with the data in our laboratory: all 83 triploid partial moles analyzed for parental origin are consistent with diandry, and in 69 of them digyny is positively ruled out. Lawler et al. [17] reported seven cases of partial moles all having two sets of paternal chromosomes.

The mechanism leading to the development of a complete mole in the presence of only paternal chromosomes and of a partial mole in the presence of excess paternal over maternal chromosomes remains unknown. It will be of interest to see if further analysis of partial moles will strengthen the correlation between the partially molar placenta and the parental origin of the extra set of chromosomes.

SUMMARY

The cytogenetic, biochemical, and RFLP data collected to date strengthen the hypothesis that complete moles have only paternal chromosomes, and the presence of only the paternal genome in some unknown way is responsible for the complete molar phenotype. In triploid partial moles the extra haploid set of chromosomes is almost always of paternal origin, and in nonmolar triploids the extra set of chromosomes is of maternal origin. Presence of one set of maternal chromosomes dilutes the molar phenotype to a partial mole. The two tetraploid partial moles in our series (92,XXXY) have three haploid paternal sets and one haploid maternal set. What distinguishes them from the normally triploid partial moles is the triandric, instead of the usual diandric, status in the presence of one maternal haploid set. This suggests that the formation of the mole is associated with an excess of paternal over maternal haploid contributions.

The clinical data confirm the well known association of complete moles and choriocarcinoma. Partial moles very rarely are capable of developing into residual trophoblastic disease, and no case of histologically proved choriocarcinoma following a partial mole has been documented to date. Considering the high incidence of partial mole, the absence of authenticated cases of carcinoma speaks for essential benignity of the condition. Of our 295 cases of partial mole, only four cases were treated with chemotherapy because hCG levels did not return to normal.

ACKNOWLEDGMENT

The above work was partially funded by NIH grant HD17572.

REFERENCES

1. Barton SC, Surani MAH, Norris ML: Role of paternal and maternal genomes in mouse development. Nature 311: 374–376, 1984.
2. Bergsma D: Cytogenetics and Cell Genetics, Vol 21, No. 6. Karger, Basel, 1978, pp. 358–362.
3. Botstein D, White RL, Skolnick M, et al.: Construction of a genetic linkage map in man using restriction fragment length polymorphisms. Am J Hum Genet 32: 314–331, 1980.
4. Couillin P, Hors J, Boué J, Boué A: Identification of the origin of triploidy by HLA markers. Hum Genet 41: 34–45, 1978.
5. Davis JR, Surwit EA, Garry JP, Fortier KJ: Sex assignment in gestational trophoblastic neoplasia. Am J Obstet Gynecol 148: 722–729, 1984.
6. Edward JLH, Yuncken C, Rushton DI, et al.: Three cases of triploidy in man. Cytogenetics 6: 81, 1967.
7. Jacobs PA, Wilson CM, Sprenkle JA, et al.: Mechanism of origin of complete hydatidiform moles. Nature 286: 714–716, 1980.

8. Jacobs PA, Angell RR, Buchanan IM, Hassold TJ: The origin of human triploids. Ann Hum Genet 42: 49–57, 1978.
9. Jacobs PA, Szulman AE, Funkhauser J, et al.: Human triploidy: Relationship between parental origin of the additional haploid complement and development of partial hydatidiform mole. Ann Hum Genet 46: 223–231, 1982.
10. Kajii T, Niikawa N: Origin of triploidy and tetraploidy in man: 11 cases with chromosome markers. Cytogenet Cell Genet 18: 109–125, 1977.
11. Kajii T, Ohama K: Androgenetic origin of hydatidiform mole. Nature 268: 633–634, 1977.
12. Kajii T: Androgenetic origin of hydatidiform moles: Its bearing on carcinogenesis. Gann Monogr Cancer Res 25: 189–194, 1980.
13. Kajii T, Kurashige H, Ohama K, Uchino F: XY and XX complete moles: Clinical and morphologic correlations. Am J Obstet Gynecol 150: 57–64, 1984.
14. Lauritsen JG: Aetiology of spontaneous abortion. A cytogenetic and epidemiological study of 288 abortuses and their parents. Acta Obstet Gynecol Scand [Suppl] 52: 2–29, 1976.
15. Lawler SD: Genetic studies on hydatidiform moles. In Pattillo RA, Hussa RO (eds): Human Trophoblastic Neoplasms. Plenum, New York, 1984, pp. 147–161.
16. Lawler SD, Povey S, Fisher RA, et al.: Genetic studies on hydatidiform moles. II. The origin of complete moles. Ann Hum Genet 46: 209, 1982.
17. Lawler SD, Fisher RA, Pickthall VJ, et al.: Genetic studies on hydatidiform moles 1. The origin of partial moles. Cancer Genet Cytogenet 5: 309–320, 1982.
18. Ohama K, Kajii T, Okamoto E, et al.: Dispermic origin of XY hydatidiform moles. Nature 292: 551–552, 1981.
19. Ojaifo J, Habibian, Surti U: Sex chromatin study of gestational trophoblastic disease. (in press).
20. Park WW: Choriocarcinoma: A study of its pathology. FA Davis, Philadelphia, 1971.
21. Surti U, Szulman AE, O'Brien S: Complete hydatidiform mole with 46,XY karyotype of paternal origin. Human Genet 51: 153–155, 1979.
22. Surti U, Szulman AE, O'Brien S: Dispermic origin and clinical outcome of three complete hydatidiform moles with 46,XY karyotype. Am J Obstet Gynecol 144: 84–87, 1982.
23. Surti U, Szulman AE, Wagner K, et al.: Tetraploid partial hydatidiform moles: Two cases with a triple paternal contribution and a 92,XXXY karyotype. Hum Genet 72: 15–21, 1986.
24. Szulman AE, Surti U: The syndromes of hydatidiform mole: 1. Cytogenetic and morphologic correlations. Am J Obstet Gynecol 131: 665–671, 1978.
25. Szulman AE, Surti U: The syndromes of hydatidiform mole: 2. Morphologic evolution. Am J Obstet Gynecol 132: 20–27, 1978.
26. Szulman AE, Phillippe E, Boué JG, Boué A: Human triploidy: Association with partial hydatidiform moles and non-molar conceptuses. Hum Pathol 12: 1016–1021, 1981.
27. Szulman AE, Surti U: The syndromes of hydatidiform mole. 3. The clinicopathological profile of the partial mole. Obstet Gynecol 59: 597–602, 1982.
28. Szulman AE, Surti U: Complete and partial hydatidiform moles: Cytogenetic and morphological aspects. In Pattilo R (ed): Human Trophoblast Neoplasm (Advances in Experimental Biology and Medicine Series). Plenum, New York, 1984.
29. Wallace DC, Surti U, Adams CW, Szulman AE: Complete moles have paternal chromosomes but maternal mitochondrial DNA. Hum Genet 61: 145–147, 1982.
30. Wake N, Takagi N, Sasaki M: Androgenesis as a cause of hydatidiform mole. J Natl Cancer Inst 60: 51, 1978.
31. Wake N, Seki T, Fujita H, et al.: Malignant potential of homozygous and heterozygous complete moles. Cancer Res 44: 1226–1230, 1984.
32. White R: In Cairns J (ed): Branbury Report 4. Cancer in Defined Populations. Cold Spring Harbor, New York, 1980, pp. 409–420.
33. Yamashita K, Wake N, Araki T, et al.: A further HLA study of hydatidiform moles. Gynecol Oncol 11: 23–28, 1981.
34. Gestational Trophoblastic Disease, Report of a WHO Scientific Group, World Health Organization, Geneva, 1983.

3

Genetic Aspects of Gestational Trophoblastic Tumors

Sylvia D. Lawler and Rosemary A. Fisher

INTRODUCTION

In 1983 a World Health Organization Scientific Group met to discuss gestational trophoblastic disease (GTD) and suggested that GTD should be used as a general clinical term to cover hydatidiform mole, invasive mole, placental site trophoblastic tumor (PSTT), and choriocarcinoma [43]. Thus GTD embraces both malignant and nonmalignant conditions. The PSTT, a malignant tumor composed of cytotrophoblast [9], occurs after term pregnancies or nonmolar abortions. No genetic studies have yet been reported for this tumor. However, the other gestational trophoblastic tumors (GTT)—i.e., nonmalignant invasive mole and malignant choriocarcinoma—have been the subject of genetic studies directed toward examining them for karyotypic abnormalities and determining the parental origin of their genome [14, 15, 27, 31, 34, 39].

In cancer cells, chromosomal changes may result in alterations in gene dosage if whole chromosomes or parts of chromosomes are gained by duplication or lost through deletion. Translocations involving balanced exchanges of chromosomal material may not result in the loss of genetic information, but they may promote the activity of protooncogenes and thus cause alterations in cell behavior characteristic of the malignant phenotype.

As well as structural changes at the chromosomal level, the malignant phenotype may be associated with particular genotypes. These can be identified by various methods including studies of restriction fragment length polymorphisms (RFLP) of the DNA. The association of a rare pattern for two polymorphic sites close to the gene for the subunit of human chorionic gonadotropin (hCG) with choriocarcinomas that follow molar pregnancies has been suggested [16].

As hydatidiform mole is an identifiable state predisposing to invasive mole or choriocarcinoma, prospective studies can be used to identify factors that increase the risk of development of a trophoblastic tumor. Factors that may be important include the pathological type and genetic origin of the mole. Partial moles are triploid, have a maternal contribution, generally have two paternal contributions, and arise by dispermy [18, 25]. Complete moles are androgenetically derived [22] and may be homozygous, arising by fertilization of an empty egg by a sperm with a doubled haploid genome [20, 24, 26]; or they may be dispermic [28], in which case they will be heterozygous for some loci. It has been suggested that these heterozygous moles have a more malignant potential than completely homozygous moles [23, 31, 39, 40].

Risk of developing choriocarcinoma has been associated with the ABO blood group of the patient [32]. Subsequently, the risk was shown to be associated not only with the blood group of the patient, but also with that of her partner [2].

This paper describes a cytogenetic study of choriocarcinoma, and a prospective study in which the clinical outcome of patients with molar pregnancy is correlated with genetic factors such as the parental origin of the mole, the ABO blood groups of the patient and her partner, and the RFLPs associated with the hCG gene.

MATERIALS

Cytogenetic Studies of Choriocarcinoma

Four established cell lines derived from gestational choriocarcinoma were studied. Two cell lines, BeWo and Jar, were preceded by term births, whereas in E1Fa and DoSmi the antecedent pregnancy was a complete hydatidiform mole. Methods of culture and preparation of chromosomes from these cell lines is given in detail elsewhere [34]. Direct chromosome preparations from a lung metastasis of a choriocarcinoma GP grown in xenograft were also examined. In this case, the antecedent pregnancy was a spontaneous abortion of unknown sex.

Prospective Study of Hydatidiform Mole

Obstetricians practicing within a 50 mile radius of The Royal Marsden Hospital cooperated by advising us when a suspected molar pregnancy was to be terminated. Fresh molar tissue and blood from the patient and her partner were then collected whenever possible.

METHODS

The macroscopical appearance of each mole was recorded. Representative sections were examined to confirm a histological diagnosis of complete or partial mole. Culturing and preparation of chromosomes from molar tissue and parental blood were carried out as previously described [25].

Cell Ploidy

Because successful culture of molar tissue is not always possible, some samples were examined by flow cytometry to determine cell ploidy. A single cell suspension was prepared by trypsinization of the molar tissue followed by preparation and staining of the nuclei with ethidium bromide using a modification of the procedure described by Vindelov in 1977 [38]. The fluorescent intensity of the molar nuclei was compared with that of diploid controls (normal lymphocytes) using a fluorescent-activated cell sorter. More recently, staining with Distamycin/DAPI, a technique by which the heterochromatic regions of chromosomes 1, 9, and 16 show bright staining that can be identified as spots in interphase nuclei [37], was used to determine the ploidy of nuclei from molar tissue.

Chromosome Polymorphisms

Where metaphases were obtained from cultured mole cells, these were stained using C-banding [35] to examine polymorphisms of the heterochromatic regions of chromosomes 1, 9, and 16. Q-banding [11] was used to examine polymorphisms of the centromere of chromosomes 3 and 13 and the satellites on chromosomes 13, 14, 15, 21, and 22. In a small number of cases, lateral asymmetry [1] of chromosome 1 was also examined. Heteromorphisms found in molar chromosomes were then compared with banded chromosomes prepared from cultured lymphocytes from the patient and her partner. The chromosomes are described according to the International Nomenclature (ISCN) [17].

Biochemical Markers

Where tissue was available, an attempt was made to type the molar tissue and parental red blood cells for the following systems: phosphoglucomutase-1 (PGM_1), phosphogluconate dehydrogenase (PGD), acid phosphatase-1 (ACP_1), glyoxalase (GLO), adenylate kinase-1 (AK_1), esterase D (ESD), and phosphoglycolate phosphatase (PGP). Molar tissue was also tested for phosphoglucomutase-3 (PGM_3), glutamic-oxaloacetic transaminase (mitochondrial) (GOT_2), and placental alkaline phosphatase (PL). In one case only, white blood cells of the parents were examined for PGM_3. The methods used have been previously described [25, 26]. The chromosome location of the enzyme systems used is shown in Table 1.

DNA Polymorphisms

Total genomic DNA was prepared by standard methods [10]. Two cDNA probes were used to examine polymorphisms in the nuclear genome. A Y chromosome-specific probe, 48CB, was used to identify Y sequences in Eco R1 digests of DNA prepared from CHM, whereas a 3′ Hinf 1 fragment of the clone pCGα [4] was used to examine molar DNA for the Eco R1 and Hind III polymorphic restriction sites in the 3′ flanking region of the αhCG gene [16].

The RFLP of mitochondrial DNA (mtDNA) from molar tissue and parental white blood cells were examined using clones pMM 4, 7, and 29 [10].

Table 1. Chromosome location of enzyme systems used

Enzyme locus	Chromosome and arm
PGM_1	1p
PGD	1p
ACP_1	2p
GLO	6p
PGM_3	6q
AK_1	9q
ESD	13q
PGP	16p
GOT_2	16q
PL	Unknown

RESULTS

Cytogenetic Studies in Chriocarcinoma

The modal chromosome numbers and sex chromosome complement of the cell lines studied are shown in Table 2. The chromosomes involved in consistent rearrangements in the four cell lines are given in Table 3. These have been described in detail elsewhere [34]. All the cell lines showed involvement of chromosomes 1 and 9 in structural rearrangements; however the breakpoints involved were different in the four cell lines (Figure 1).

Few analyzable cells were found in the tumor GP. Complete metaphases had 47 chromosomes, the additional chromosome involving part of a number 1 chromosome,

Table 2. Chromosome numbers and sex chromosome complement of 4 choriocarcinoma cell lines

Cell line	No. of cells examined	Chromosome number		Sex chromosome complement
		Range	Mode	
BeWo	63	55–89	75	XY
Jar	78	59–84	74/76	XXYor i(Xq)Y
ElFa	45	61–91	80	XY
DoSmi	50	61–89	81	X

Table 3. Chromosomes involved in structural rearrangements in 4 choriocarcinoma cell lines

Cell line	Chromosomes						
BeWo	1	6	7	9	13	22	
Jar	1	4	9	12	16	X	
ElFa	1	4	7	9	10	12	14
DoSmi	1	9	11	22			

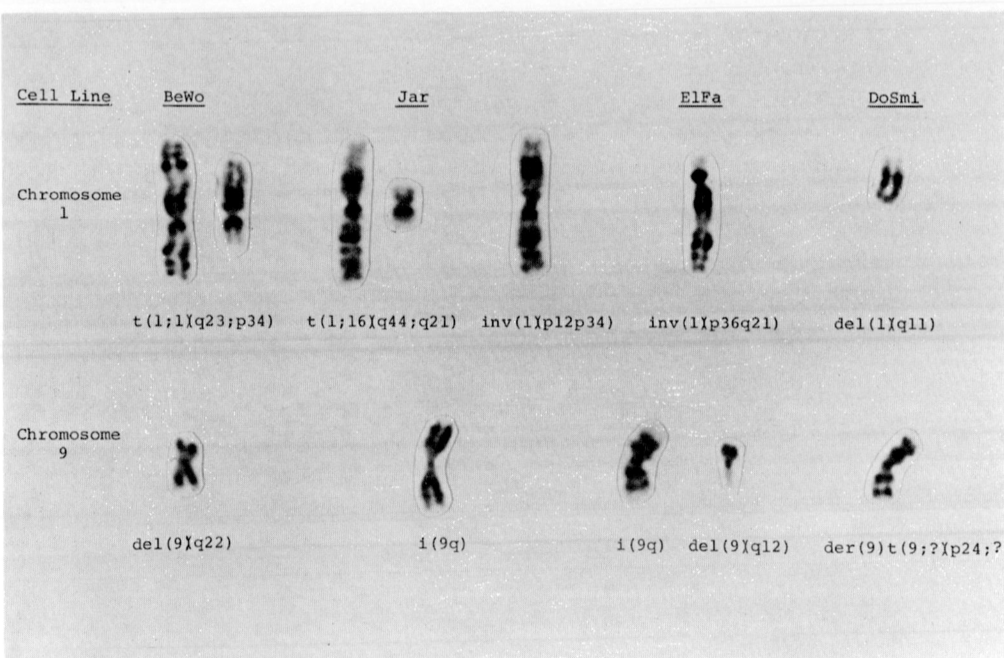

Figure 1. Rearrangements in choriocarcinoma cell lines involving chromosome number 1 or chromosome number 9.

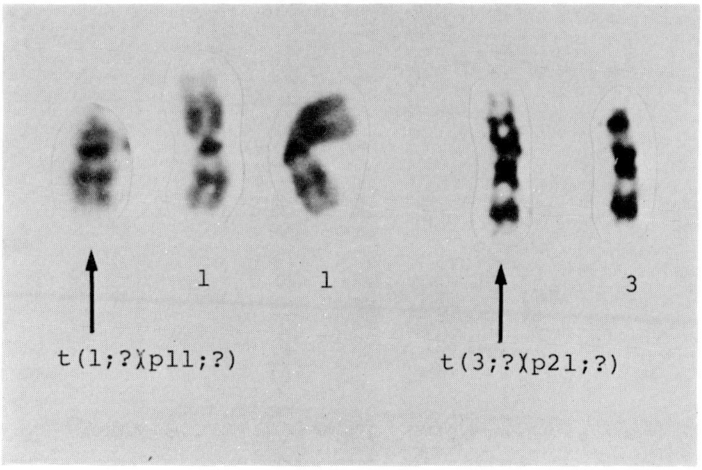

Figure 2. Structural chromosome abnormalities in choriocarcinoma GP.

t (1; ?) (p11; ?). A consistent rearrangement of one number 3 chromosome t (3; ?) (p21; ?) was also identified (Figure 2).

Examination of the sex chromosome complement of the cells lines showed that three of them had both X and Y chromosomes present, indicating that they were, in fact, heterozygous. A Y chromosome was not identified in the DoSmi cell line, whereas the tumor GP was found to have two X chromosomes in those cells that could be analyzed. In the DoSmi cell line, heteromorphism of the centromeric regions of the number 3 chromosomes and the satellites on the number 21 chromosomes showed that this line was also heterozygous in origin. The tumor GP showed heteromorphisms of the number 1 and 9 chromosomes when C-banded.

Prospective Study of Hydatidiform Mole

As of March 1985, 150 hydatidiform moles had been entered in the study on the basis of a pathological diagnosis.

Partial hydatidiform mole. On the basis of pathology, 36 hydatidiform moles were diagnosed as partial. Triploidy was demonstrated in some cases by flow cytometry or DA/DAPI staining. In 24 cases examined, the partial hydatidiform moles (PHM) were found to have chromosome numbers in the triploid range. Where the karyotype was successfully determined, 9 were found to be 69,XXY; 10 were found to be 69,XXX; one was 71,XXY, having two additional C group chromosomes; and one was 70,XXY, with a marker derived from a number 15 chromosome. The genetic origin could be deduced in 20 of the PHM and in all cases was compatible with a single maternal contribution and two paternal contributions to the genome. An origin by dispermy was possible in all 20 cases and was proved in 14. In all cases of PHM there was a spontaneous resolution of the pregnancy after the evacuation of the mole. None of the patients required subsequent chemotherapy.

Complete hydatidiform mole. Of 114 hydatidiform moles were classified as complete, 21 (18%) subsequently required treatment for GTT.

1. Genetic origin of complete hydatidiform moles. All complete hydatidiform moles (CHM) for which the karyotype was determined were found to be diploid.

In 74 cases chromosomal and biochemical markers were examined. In 67 cases all markers studied were homozygous, whereas in seven cases there was evidence of heterozygosity. Of these, seven CHM, one was 46,XX; five were 46,XY; and one was Y-body positive.

The requirement for treatment in relation to the genetic type of the CHM is summarized in Table 4. The frequency with which treatment was required after evacuation of

Table 4. Summary of genetic studies in 114 cases of complete mole

	No. of cases with no further treatment after evacuation	No. of cases having chemotherapy after evacuation
Total	93	21 (18%)
Tested for genetic markers	60	14
Homozygous moles	55	12 (18%)
Heterozygous moles	5	2 (29%)

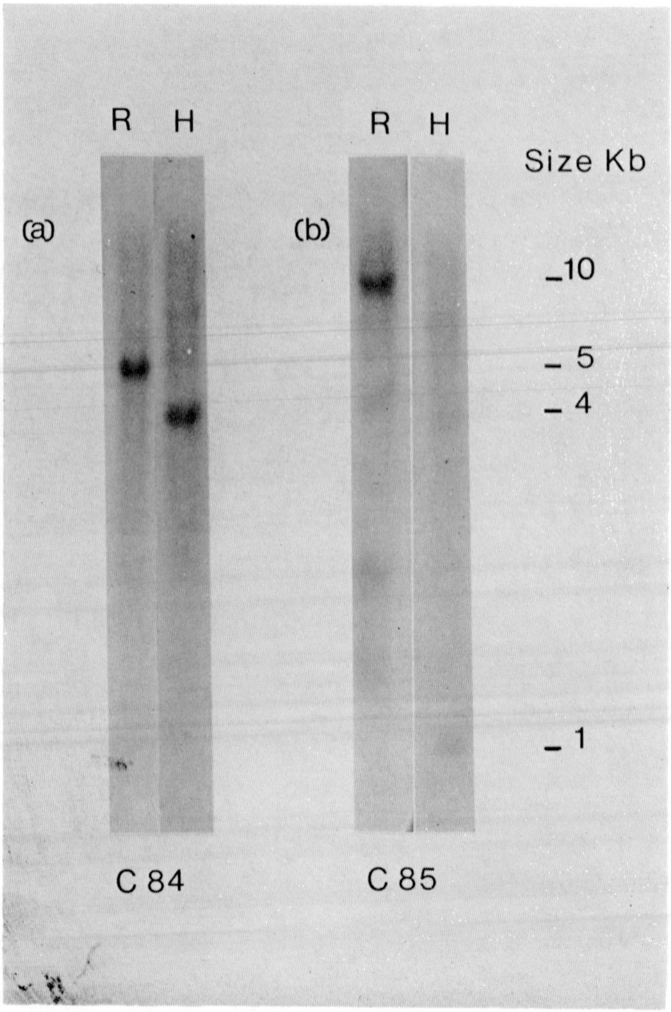

Figure 3. Restriction fragments of Eco R1 (R) and Hind III (H) digests of DNA from CHM, hybridized to a 3′ Hinf 1 fragment of the hCG α clone. (a) C84 shows the pattern generated by presence of the Eco R1 and the absence of the Hind III site, R^+H^-/R^+H^-, (b) C85 shows pattern generated by presence of the Hind III and the absence of the Eco R1 site, R^-H^+/R^-H^+.

Table 5. ABO blood groups in patients with complete mole*

ABO mating type	Outcome after evacuation of mole		Total
	Spontaneous resolution	Chemotherapy required	
Like	25	0	25
Unlike	44	19	63
Total	69	19	88

* $p=0.001$.

CHM was higher in those classified as heterozygous (29%) than in those classified as homozygous (18%).

The mitochondrial genome was examined in 27 CHM by analyzing the restriction fragments generated by 13 different restriction enzymes. Seven variant patterns were found in six CHM, one of which did not resolve spontaneously after treatment. No unusual variants were found in any of the CHM studied, and all morphisms found had been previously described [6, 7, 21].

Examination of RFLP in the mtDNA of the parents of the CHM with variant patterns showed that in each case the variant pattern was found in the patient's DNA. Therefore the mtDNA in molar tissue was maternally inherited.

2. RFLP associated with the αhCG gene. Seven homozygous CHM were tested for the Eco R1 and Hind III polymorphisms. Three cases were found to have the diplotype R^+H^-/R^+H^- and four to be R^-H^+/R^-H^+ (Figure 3). One patient in each category required treatment.

3. ABO blood groups in the parents of complete hydatidiform moles. The mating types of the parents of the CHMs were classified as like matings if the blood groups of the parents were A×A, O×O, B×B, or AB×AB. All other matings were in the unlike category. Spontaneous resolution was highly correlated with like mating type (Table 5).

DISCUSSION

Cytogenetic Studies of Choriocarcinoma

All karyotypes in choriocarcinomas reported so far have shown both numerical and structural abnormalities. This applies not only to cell lines [31, 33, 34] where karyotypic evolution may have taken place, but also to tumors grown in xenograft [14, 39].

All four cell lines studied showed rearrangements of chromosomes number 1 and 9; however, the arrangements involved different breakpoints in each of the lines. The tumor GP showed a number 1 chromosome with the breakpoint at p11, which is near the location of the *NRAS* protooncogene, 1p11–13 [30]. This rearrangement made the tumor effectively trisomic for 1q, and it is of interest that two of three tumors described by Wake et al. [39] had a gain of material from 1q. However, rearrangements of chromosome number 1 are frequently seen in solid tumors, particularly those involving breakpoints near the centromere [5].

Although the karyotypes of few choriocarcinomas have been determined, sex has been determined by Y-body staining of tissue sections. In a study by Davis et al. [8], 14 of 19 specimens were found to be Y-body positive. Among choriocarcinomas following term births, an approximately equal number of XX and XY tumors would be expected. However, because the majority of CHM are XX, in choriocarcinoma after CHM a predominance of XX might be expected. Although the antecedent pregnancy was not defined by Davis et al. [8], their data nevertheless indicate an excess of XY in histologically proved choriocarcinomas. The small number of tumors studied cytogenetically have yielded an approximately equal number of tumors with or without a Y chromosome [14, 31, 33, 34, 39]. Studies of chromosome polymorphisms in choriocarcinomas have shown that, whether the choriocarcinoma tissue or cell lines studied were preceded by term births, nonmolar abortions, or CHM, they have all been heterozygous for some genetic loci, demonstrated either by a Y chromosome or by heteromorphic autosomes. This observation is consistent with the suggestion that heterozygous CHM have more malignant potential than those with a doubled haploid genome.

Prospective Study of Hydatidiform Mole

Partial hydatidiform mole. The proportion of PHM to CHM in any series of patients depends on the method of ascertainment. If the patients are selected because hydatidiform mole is suspected, then a lower proportion (24% in this series) will be found than if the series is composed of patients who, for example, have had a spontaneous abortion. In such a series, Jacobs et al. [19] diagnosed 69% to be PHM.

In our series all 36 PHM resolved spontaneously. It therefore appears that PHM is rarely followed by GTT, and it is suggested that the risk of GTT after PHM may not be greater than after a normal conception. In cases where the possibility of PHM requiring treatment is suggested, care must be taken to exclude the presence of CHM with non-identical twin [12] and to ensure that the pregnancy with PHM is causally related to the tumor.

Complete hydatidiform mole. Among the 114 CHM, 24 (18%) did not resolve spontaneously. Of these, two of seven proved heterozygous CHM required chemotherapy for a clinically diagnosed trophoblastic tumor. Although the numbers are small, the findings support the contention that heterozygous CHM are at greater risk for development of GTT than homozygous CHM. Of the 81 CHM tested for genetic markers in our series, 7 (8.8%) were heterozygous. There are problems distinguishing between homozygous and heterozygous CHM because the latter are heterozygous at some loci but homozygous at others. Furthermore, only loci for which the male parent is heterozygous are informative. If a Y chromosome is present, it can be readily detected by Y-body staining or at the DNA level by the use of Y-specific probes (Figure 4). Where a CHM is 46, XX, an adequate number of autosomal polymorphisms for which the father is heterozygous must be studied in order to minimize the possibility of missing a heterozygous CHM. The most likely mechanism of origin of heterozygous CHM is by dispermy [13, 28, 29, 36]. Statistically, to exclude the possibility at the 95% confidence level of a CHM being dispermic, at least five informative polymorphisms on different chromosomes should be examined. The possibility of heterozygous CHM arising by a failure of meiosis II must be borne in mind, and it may be necessary to examine more polymorphisms to detect this.

The cells of CHM are unique in that the nuclear genome is paternal and the mitochondrial genome maternal [10, 41]. The risk of developing GTT after CHM has not yet been related to any particular mitochondrial genome [10].

In a search for other factors influencing the risk of choriocarcinoma developing after CHM, we have made a preliminary study of the polymorphic sites in the region of the αhCG gene. Hoshina et al. [16] found that 10 of 12 CHM belonged to the common diplotype R^+H^-/R^+H^-, whereas three of four choriocarcinomas that followed CHM were of the rare diplotype R^-H^+/R^-H^+. They suggested that hydatidiform moles that were likely to progress to choriocarcinoma would have the rare diplotype. In our small series of CHM we found an equal distribution between the two diplotypes, whereas one CHM

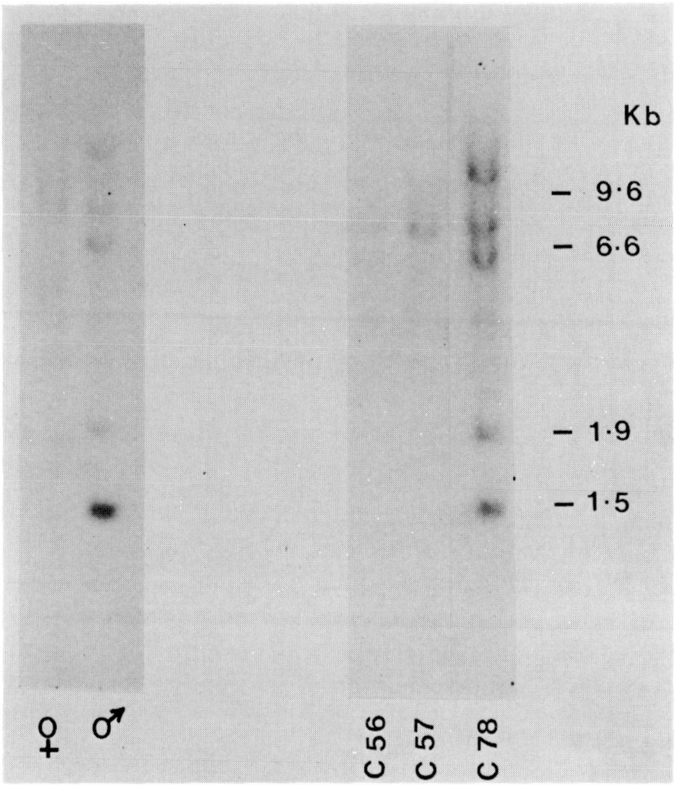

Figure 4. Restriction fragments from Eco R1 digests of DNA hybridized to the 48CB clone showing differential patterns in DNA from male (♂) and female (♀) white blood cells. DNA from CHM C56, karyotype 46,XX, shows the female pattern; whereas C78, karyotype 46,XY, shows the male specific bands; C57, of unknown karyotype, shows the female pattern of hybridization.

in each group progressed to GTT. Further prospective studies are clearly required to evaluate the risk factor associated with various diplotypes for these polymorphisms.

There has been much interest for many years in the ABO blood group frequency in patients with choriocarcinoma. In 1962 Scott [32] found a decrease of blood group O patients in a series of patients collected in the USA. Subsequently Bagshawe et al. [2] showed that the risk of a patient developing choriocarcinoma depends not only on the ABO group of the patient, but also on that of her partner. A study of 115 cases of choriocarcinoma after a normal conceptus studied in the UK showed a relative risk of 2.19 for the patient and partner matings

$$\frac{A \times O + O \times A}{A \times A + O \times O},$$

where the control value was 1.0 [3]. In our series of CHM, we found a very strong influence of the ABO mating type such that when patient and partner have the same blood group, the risk of development of GTT is reduced.

Our data suggest that an ABO incompatible environment favors trophoblastic proliferation. However, because of the androgenetic origin of the CHM, a mating that is scored as unlike—for example, O (mother) × A (father)—may produce a conceptus that is like the mother if the male parent is heterozygous AO and a group O type sperm duplicates. Similarly a mating scored as like may result in a conceptus unlike the mother.

The ABO blood groups are not expressed on the trophoblast in sufficient quantity to be detected by current immunohistopathological techniques. The expression of ABO blood groups on cell membranes depends on the addition of sugars to precursor oligosaccharides by glycosyl transferases, which are the products of the A and B genes [42]. Lack of expression of the antigen may be due to a lack of precursors or to the effect of other regulator genes. The presence of precursors can be determined by estimating A and B transferases; a collaborative study is now in progress.

An effect of the ABO group in GTT has been demonstrated, but the mechanism is at present obscure and merits further study.

ACKNOWLEDGMENTS

The biochemical marker and DNA studies were carried out in collaboration with Dr. S. Povey, Dr. Y. Edwards, and S. Jeremiah of the MRC Biochemical Genetics Unit, London. We express our thanks to Dr. R. Pattillo for donating the cell lines examined, and to Professor K. D. Bagshawe for supplying the tumor GP. We are also grateful to D. M. Sheppard, D. Rowe, and E. J. Maher for help with determining the karyotypes. The probes used in the DNA studies were kindly donated by Dr. C. Bishop (48CB), Dr. I. Boime (pCGα), and Dr. I. Craig (pMM 4, 7, 29). This work was supported by a Medical Research Council grant to the Fetal Tissue Bank and the joint Medical Research Council/Cancer Research Campaign funding of the Section of Human Genetics.

REFERENCES

1. Angel RR, Jacobs PA: Lateral asymmetry in human constitutive heterochromatin. Frequency and inheritance. Am J Hum Genet 30: 144–152, 1978.
2. Bagshawe KD, Rawlins G, Pike MC, et al.: ABO blood-groups in trophoblastic neoplasia. Lancet i: 553–557, 1971.
3. Bagshawe KD: Some facets of trophoblastic neoplasia in man. J Reprod Fertil [Suppl] 31: 175–179, 1982.
4. Boothby M, Ruddon RW, Anderson C, et al.: A single gonadotropin-subunit gene in normal tissue and tumor-derived cell lines. J Biol Chem 256: 5121–5127, 1981.
5. Brito-Babapulle V, Atkin NB: Break points in chromosome number 1. Abnormalities of 218 human neoplasms. Cancer Genet Cytogenet 4: 215–225, 1981.
6. Brown WM, Goodman HM: Quantitation of intrapopulation variation by restriction endonuclease analysis of human mitochondrial DNA. In Cummings DJ, Borst P, et al. (eds): Extrachromosomal DNA. Academic Press, London, 1979, pp. 485–499.
7. Brown WM: Polymorphism in mitochondrial DNA of humans as revealed by restriction endonuclease analysis. Proc Natl Acad Sci 77: 3605–3609, 1980.
8. Davis JR, Surwit EA, Perada J, et al.: Sex assignment in gestational trophoblastic neoplasia. Am J Obstet Gynecol 148: 722–725, 1984.
9. Eckstein RP, Paradinas FJ, Bagshawe KD: Placental site trophoblastic tumour (trophoblastic pseudotumour): A study of four cases requiring hysterectomy including one fatal case. Histopathology 6: 211–226, 1982.
10. Edwards YH, Jeremiah SJ, McMillan SL, et al.: Complete hydatidiform moles combine maternal mitochondria with a paternal nuclear genome. Ann Hum Genet 48: 119–127, 1984.
11. Evans HJ, Buckton KE, Summer AT: Cytological mapping of human chromosomes: Results obtained with quinacrine fluorescence and the acetic-saline-Giemsa technique. Chromosoma (Berlin) 35: 310–325, 1971.
12. Fisher RA, Sheppard DM, Lawler SD: Twin pregnancy with complete hydatidiform mole (46,XX) and fetus (46,XY): Genetic origin proved by analysis of chromosome polymorphisms. Br Med J 284: 1218–1220, 1982.
13. Fisher RA, Sheppard DM, Lawler SD: Two patients with complete mole with 46,XX karyotype. Br J Obstet Gynaecol 91: 690–693, 1984.

14. Fisher RA, Sheppard DM, Lawler SD: Cytogenetics of gestational choriocarcinomas. In Proceedings of the Second World Congress on Trophoblastic Neoplasms. (in press).
15. Galton M, Goldman PB, Holt SF: Karyotypic and morphological characterisation of a serially transplanted human choriocarcinoma. J Natl Cancer Inst 31: 1019–1035, 1963.
16. Hoshina M, Boothby MR, Hussa RD, et al.: Segregation patterns of polymorphic restriction sites of the gene encoding the α subunit of human chorionic gonadotropin in trophoblastic disease. Proc Natl Acad Sci 81: 2504–2507, 1984.
17. ISCN: An international system for human cytogenetic nomenclature, 1978. Cytogenet Cell Genet 21: 309–404, 1978.
18. Jacobs PA, Szulman AE, Funkhouser J, et al.: Human triploidy: Relationship between parental origin of the additional haploid complement and development of partial hydatidiform mole. Ann Hum Genet 46: 223–231, 1982.
19. Jacobs PA, Hunt PA, Matsuura JS, et al.: Complete and partial hydatidiform mole in Hawaii: Cytogenetics, morphology and epidemiology. Br J Obstet Gynaecol 89: 256–266, 1982.
20. Jacobs RA, Wilson CM, Sprenkle JA, et al.: Mechanism of origin of complete hydatidiform moles. Nature 286: 714–716, 1980.
21. Johnson MJ, Wallace DC, Ferris SD, et al.: Radiation of human mitochondrial DNA types analysed by restriction endonuclease cleavage patterns. J Mol Evol 19: 255–271, 1983.
22. Kajii T, Ohama K: Androgenetic origin of hydatidiform mole. Nature 268: 633–634, 1977.
23. Kajii T: Androgenetic origin of hydatidiform moles: Its bearing on carcinogenesis. Gann Monogr Cancer Res 25: 189–194, 1980.
24. Lawler SD, Pickthall VJ, Fisher RA, et al.: Genetic studies of complete and partial hydatidiform moles. Lancet ii: 580, 1979.
25. Lawler SD, Fisher RA, Pickthall VJ, et al.: Genetic studies on hydatidiform moles. I. The origin of partial moles. Cancer Genet Cytogenet 5: 309–320, 1982.
26. Lawler SD, Povey S, Fisher RA, et al.: Genetic studies on hydatidiform moles. II. The origin of complete moles. Ann Hum Genet 46: 209–222, 1982.
27. Makino S, Sasaki MS, FukuschimaT: Cytological studies of tumors XLI, chromosomal instability in human chorionic lesions. Okajimas Fol Anat Jpn 40: 439–465, 1965.
28. Ohama K, Kajii T, Okamoto E, et al.: Dispermic origin of XY hydatidiform moles. Nature 29: 551–552, 1981.
29. Patillo RA, Sasaki S, Katayama KP, et al.: Genesis of 46,XY hydatidiform mole. Am J Obstet Gynecol 141: 104–105, 1981.
30. Rabin M, Watson M, Barker PE, et al.: *NRAS* transforming gene maps to region p11→p13 on chromosome 1 by in situ hybridization. Cytogenet Cell Genet 38: 70–72, 1984.
31. Sasaki S, Katayama PK, Roesler M, et al.: Cytogenetic analysis of choriocarcinoma cell lines. Acta Obstet Gynaecol Jpn 34: 2253–2256, 1982.
32. Scott JS: Choriocarcinoma; observations on the etiology. Am J Obstet Gynecol 83: 185–193, 1962.
33. Sekiya S, Shirotake S, Kaiho T, et al.: A newly established human gestational choriocarcinoma cell line and its characterization. Gynecol Oncol 15: 413–421, 1983.
34. Sheppard DM, Fisher RA, Lawler SD: Karyotypic analysis and chromosome polymorphisms in four choriocarcinoma cell lines. Cancer Genet Cytogenet 16: 251–259, 1985.
35. Sumner AT: A simple technique for demonstrating centromeric heterochromatin. Exp Cell Res 75: 304–306, 1972.
36. Surti U, Szulman AE, O'Brien S: Dispermic origin and clinical outcome of three complete hydatidiform moles with 46,XY karyotype. Am J Obstet Gynecol 144: 84–87, 1982.
37. Tommerup N, Vejerslev LO: Identification of triploidy by DA/DAPI staining of trophoblastic interphase nuclei. Placenta (in press).
38. Vindelov L: Flow microfluorometric analysis of nuclear DNA in cells from solid tumors and cell suspensions. Virchows Arch [Cell Pathol] 24: 227–242, 1977.
39. Wake N, Tanaka K-I, Chapman V, et al.: Chromosomes and cellular origin of choriocarcinoma. Cancer Res 41: 3137–3143, 1981.
40. Wake N, Seki T, Fujita H, et al.: Malignant potential of homozygous and heterozygous complete moles. Cancer Res 44: 1226–1230, 1984.
41. Wallace DC, Surti U, Adams C, et al.: Complete moles have paternal chromosomes but maternal mitochondrial DNA. Hum Genet 61: 145–147, 1982.
42. Watkins WM, Yates AD, Greenwell P: Blood group antigens and the enzymes involved in their synthesis: Past and present. Biochem Soc Trans 9: 186–191, 1981.
43. WHO Scientific Group: Gestational trophoblastic disease. World Health Organisation technical report series 692, 1983.

4

Oncogene Expression in Trophoblastic Disease

Ernest I. Kohorn, Saumyendra Sarkar, Barry M. Kacinski, Karin J. Blakemore, Maria J. Merino, and Darryl Carter

INTRODUCTION

That viruses are responsible for inducing cancer in various animal species has been known for more than 50 years. However, it was only recently that the discovery of reverse transcriptase in retroviruses and recombination techniques have permitted more detailed investigation of the factors involved. It was then appreciated that the genes responsible for viral oncogenesis are very similar in structure to genes found in normal cells and particularly those in some embryonic tissue [1]. These genes, called cellular oncogenes, may be normally expressed during cell proliferation and division. In mature cells they are repressed. This repression may be absolved by the acquisition of new regulatory sequences [3, 7], by gene amplification [2], or by mutations [11, 14]. Such mechanisms lead to excess production of oncogene messenger RNA and protein, or to production of abnormally active mutant gene products. This then leads to uncontrolled cell proliferation (cell immortality) and to abnormal metabolic derangements associated with neoplasia.

Evidence is accumulating that several oncogenes need to be expressed for invasive malignancy to be induced [5, 12]. The first oncogene then causes the cell to proliferate indefinitely in culture, and the action of a second and subsequent oncogenes may be necessary for cells to become malignant [6].

The present report concerns the investigation of oncogene expression in benign and malignant trophoblast. The progression from the hypercellular state of early normal trophoblast, through hydatidiform mole, to choriocarcinoma corresponds to oncogene expression in normal tissue, in low-grade malignancy, and in frank invasive metastasizing

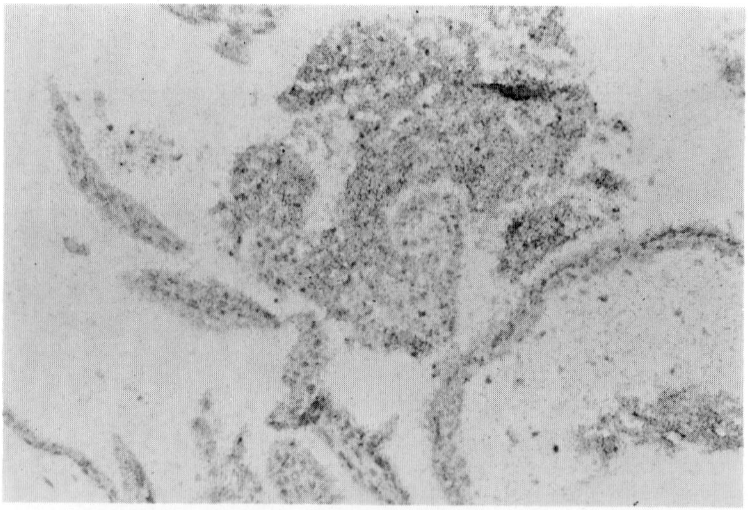

Figure 1. Seen here is c-myc oncogene expression demonstrated by in situ hybridization in the cytotrophoblast of hydatidiform mole.

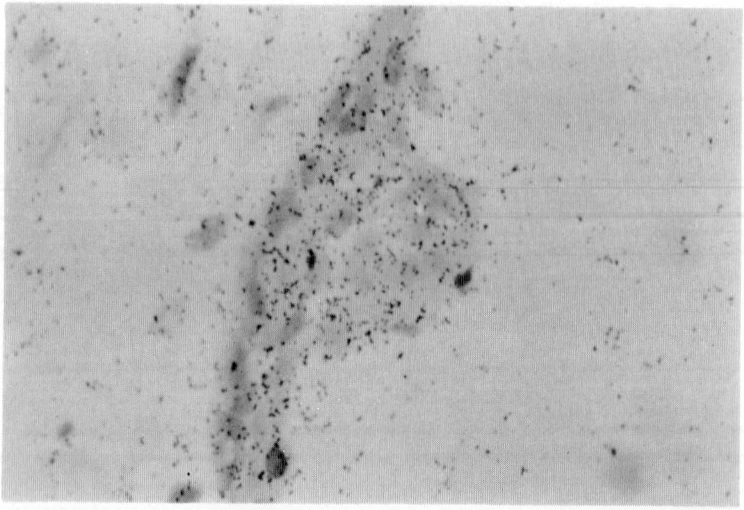

Figure 2. Cultured choriocarcinoma cell line Be-Wo (kindly supplied by Dr. Roland Patillo) to demonstrate expression of c-myc oncogene.

cancer.

We have used in situ hybridization to identify the expression of the oncogene in fixed tissue sections [8]. These are incubated with radioactively labeled probe DNA to allow hybridization of the probe with the homologous nucleic acid fixed in the specimen. ^{35}S was used to label the nucleotide because it has a ten-fold lower energy level and a smaller emulsion track length than the previously used ^{32}P.

Six hydatidiform moles have so far been examined and all demonstrated c-myc oncogene expression. This appeared to be confined to the cytotrophoblast (Figure 1). Expression of c-myc oncogene was found in early villous trophoblast at 4 weeks post-conception, and expression was not apparent at 9 weeks postconception. There was marked expression of c-myc oncogene in the malignant trophoblast cell line Be-Wo (Figure 2). There was no expression in term placenta.

DISCUSSION

Sarkar et al. [13] have demonstrated hybridization of ^{35}S-labeled myc oncogene DNA to specific cells in preimplantation rat embryos. Pfeifer-Ohlsson et al. [10], using Northern blot and in situ hybridization, have demonstrated the expression of human c-myc probes in early human villous cytotrophoblast with a peak expression at 5 weeks after conception and a decline by the end of the first trimester of pregnancy. They suggested a strong correlation between myc transcript abundance and cytotrophoblastic proliferation. More recently, Goustin et al. [4] used an in situ hybridization technique to demonstrate the expression of sis protooncogene, the structural gene for the B-chain of platelet-derived growth factor, in first trimester human cytotrophoblast.

Using the technique of in situ hybridization, we have demonstrated the expression of the cellular oncogene c-myc in the cytotrophoblast of hydatidiform mole and in the cells of the choriocarcinoma cell line Be-Wo. The expression of c-fos oncogene has previously been demonstrated by Northern blot analysis in this choriocarcinoma cell line [9]. The c-myc oncogene expression has been previously demonstrated in early normal trophoblast with lack of expression by the end of the first trimester. The present findings are thus in agreement with those of Pfeifer-Ohlsson et al. [10]. Like these investigators, we failed to demonstrate oncogene expression in term placenta.

The trophoblast of early placenta has many of the attributes of malignant tissue. It proliferates rapidly and "invades" the endometrium. Expression of certain cellular oncogenes may provide for rapid cell growth in the early trophoblast, but it is currently still unknown how this physiologic oncogene expression differs from that seen during the malignant transformation of trophoblast to invasive mole and choriocarcinoma. It is the specific aim of our further studies to determine whether there may be a particular pattern of oncogene expression characteristic of invasive neoplasia. If such a pattern can be identified, we may have found a means to identify those hydatidiform moles that may be associated with malignant sequelae.

ACKNOWLEDGMENT

This paper has been adapted from the American Journal of Obstetrics and Gynecology, volume 154, number 2, pages 390 to 393, 1986 with full permission.

REFERENCES

1. Bishop JM: Celluar oncogenes and retroviruses. Ann Rev Biochem 52: 301–354, 1983.
2. Blair DG, Oskarsson M, Wood TG, McClements WL, Fischinger PJ, Vande Woude GG: Activation of the transforming potential of a normal cell sequence: A molecular model for oncogenesis. Science 212: 941–943, 1981.
3. Collins SJ, Groudine M: Amplification of endogenous myc-related DNA sequences in a human myeloid leukemia cell line. Nature 298: 679–681, 1982.
4. Goustin AS, Betsholsz C, Pfeifer-Ohlsson S, Persson H, Rydnert J, Bywater M, Holmgren G, Heldin CH, Westermark B, Ohlsson R: Coexpression of the sis and myc proto-oncogenes in developing human placenta suggests autocrine control of trophoblast growth. Cell 41: 301–312, 1985.

5. Land H, Parada LF, Weinberg, RA: Tumorigenic conversion of primary embryo fibroblasts require at least two cooperating oncogenes. Nature 304: 596–602, 1983.
6. Land H, Parada LF, Weinberg RA: Cellular oncogenes and multistep carcinogenesis. Science 222: 771–778, 1983.
7. Leder P, Battey J, Lenoir G, Moulding C, Murphy W, Potter H, Stewart T, Taub R: Translocation among antibody genes in human cancer. Science 222: 765–771, 1983.
8. Lewin B: Gene Expression-II, 2nd ed. Wiley-Interscience, New York, 1980, pp. 517–523.
9. Muller R, Tremblay JM, Adamson ED, Verman LM: Tissue and cell type-specific expression of two human c-onc genes. Nature 304: 484–486, 1983.
10. Pfeifer-Ohlsson S, Goutsin AS, Rydnert J, Wahlstrom T, Bjersin L, Stehelin D, Ohlsson R: Spatial and temporal pattern of cellular myc oncogene expression in developing human placenta: Implications for embryonic cell proliferation. Cell 38: 585–596, 1984.
11. Reddy EP, Reynolds RK, Santos E, Barbacid M: A point mutation is responsible for the acquisition of transforming properties by the T24 human bladder carcinoma oncogene. Nature 300: 149–152, 1982.
12. Ruley EH: Adenovirus early region 1A enables viral and cellular transforming genes to transform primary cells in culture. Nature 304: 602–606, 1983.
13. Sarkar S, Maharajan V, Sanyal M, Summers WC: Myc-Gene Expression in Pre-implantation Rat Embryos. Proceedings of the Seventh International Congress of Endocrinology, Quebec, July 1984.
14. Tabin CJ, Bradley SM, Bargmann CL, Weinberg RA, Papageorge AG, Scolnick EM, Dhar R, Lowry DR, Change EH: Mechanism of activation of a human oncogene. Nature 300: 143–149, 1982.

PART TWO

IMMUNOLOGY OF TROPHOBLASTIC DISEASES

5

A Study of Cell-Mediated Immune Response in Trophoblastic Disease: With Special Reference to the Clinical Significance of Serum Immunosuppressive Effect

Tadashi Sugawa, Naohiko Umesaki, Kazutaka Hamada, and Toshitsugu Tamura

INTRODUCTION

Because human chorionic gonadotropin (hCG) is produced in trophoblastic disease, it is used as a marker for detecting malignancy sequential to hydatidiform mole and also for evaluating the efficacy of a treatment or the degree of remission of the disease condition. The importance of hCG as a tumor marker in the management of patients with trophoblastic disease is undeniable. However, this parameter alone is of little value for differentiation between choriocarcinoma and invasive mole, ascertainment of various pathological states, acquisition of prognostic information, and prediction of malignancy secondary to hydatidiform mole.

From a pathogenetic point of view, trophoblastic disease is characterized as transplanted tumor. It is presumed that immune reactions are active in patients with this disease and that the serum immunosuppressive effect in them is stronger than in normal pregnant women.

In the present investigation we studied the immunocapacity of patients with trophoblastic disease by referring to diverse blood cell factors and serum factors. The primary purpose of this study was to find a new marker that may be supplemental to hCG.

SUBJECTS

The subjects studied were patients admitted to Osaka City University Hospital for the treatment of trophoblastic diseases. Normal pregnant women in the first trimester of gestation served as controls. The patients were classified according to the diagnostic criteria established by the Japanese Obstetrical and Gynecological Association [14]. Clinical choriocarcinoma and clinical invasive mole diagnosed according to Ishizuka's score were classified as choriocarcinoma and invasive mole, respectively.

METHODS

Cell-Mediated Immune Capacity

The function of lymphocytes, especially T-cells, was studied in light of not only blood cell factors, but also serum factors that act inhibitively upon blood cell factors.

Blood cell factors. White blood cell count, lymphocyte count, T-cell count, and mononuclear cell reactivity to phytohemagglutinin (PHA) were determined. T-cells were identified by assessment of the rosette-forming capacity of sheep erythrocytes. The absolute number of T-cells was determined by multiplying the ratio of T-cells (to total lymphocytes) by the total number of lymphocytes. The reactivity of mononuclear cells to PHA was determined by our whole blood microculture method (Table 1).

Serum factors. Serum immunosuppressive effect was evaluated according to the procedure shown in Table 2 and briefly described as follows: added to normal human whole blood microculture was test serum, which was equivalent in amount to 30% of the culture medium. In a controlled experiment, normal serum was substituted for test serum.

Table 1. Micromethod using whole blood culture for evaluating cellular immune response

1. Peripheral blood collected with a heparinized syringe
2. Mixture of 0.05 mL heparinized whole blood and 0.95 mL RPMI-1640 containing 20μg PHA-P (Difco)
3. Incubation at 37°C for 24 hr in the CO_2-chamber
4. ^{3}H-thymidine (1 μCi/tube) added
5. Additional 24 hr incubation at 37°C in the CO_2-chamber
6. Erythrocytes lysed with about 3 ml distilled water
7. Lymphocytes trapped on the membrane filter
8. Uptake of ^{3}H-thymidine assessed by scintillation counter

Table 2. Immunosuppressive effect of serum on mononuclear cell mononuclear cell response to PHA

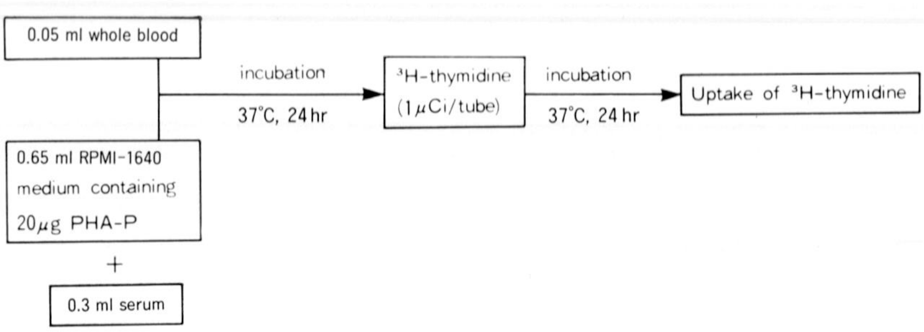

% Inhibition

$$= 100 - \frac{\Delta \text{ cpm (treated by serum from patient)}}{\Delta \text{ cpm (treated by control serum)}} \times 100$$

The inhibitory effect of the serum on normal mononuclear cell response to PHA was expressed in terms of percent inhibition.

Immunosuppressive acidic protein (IAP), one of the immunosuppressive factors in serum, was measured by the single immunodiffusion using the IAP plate (Kaken Antibiotics Co.) [15].

RESULTS

Cell-Mediated Immune Capacity

Blood cell factors (*Table 3*). In the choriocarcinoma group, leukocyte count, lymphocyte count, and mononuclear cell reactivity to PHA were decreased. However, no statistically significant differences were observed between the individual groups including the normal pregnancy group, with respect to any blood cell factor.

Serum factors (*Figure 1*)

1. Serum immunosuppressive effect. The serum immunosuppressive effect was significantly greater in the choriocarcinoma group than in the invasive mole group ($p<0.10$) or the hydatidiform mole group ($p<0.01$), but did not significantly differ between the invasive mole group and the hydatidiform mole group. Comparison between each

Table 3. Cellular immune capacity of patients with trophoblastic disease

Parameter	Diseases			Pregnancy (2–3 gest. mo)
	Hydatidiform	Invasive mole	Choriocarcinoma	
WBC/mm^3	5,918±1,891	6,173±2,227	5,544±1,618	6,600±1,700
Lymphocyte count/mm^3	2,045±681	1,870±718	1,557±689	1,800±500
T-cell count/mm^3	1,612±530	1,375±531	1,390±742	1,400±150
Mononuclear cell reactivity to PHA (cpm)	37,500±11,500	36,248±13,995	32,290±13,940	34,000±10,000

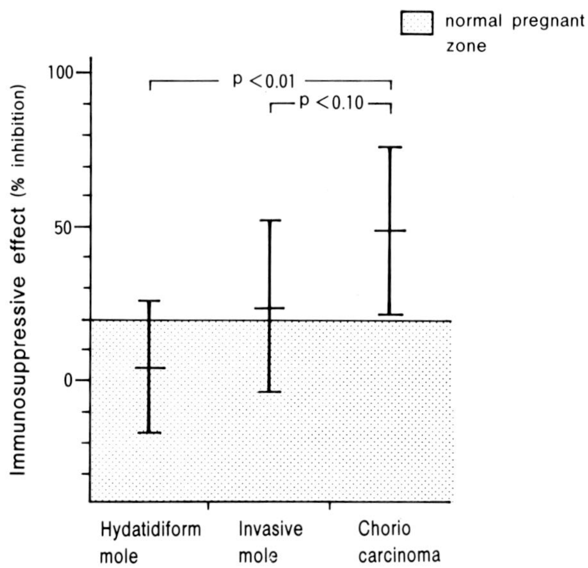

Figure 1. Serum immunosuppressive effect in trophoblastic diseases.

disease group and the normal pregnancy group disclosed no significant difference except between the choriocarcinoma group and the normal pregnancy group ($p<0.01$).

2. IAP level (Figure 2). Given that cases with an IAP level higher than 500 μg/mL are positive, only the choriocarcinoma group was positive when judged on the basis of the mean IAP level. The IAP level (mean±S.D.) in the choriocarcinoma group was significantly higher than that in the invasive mole group ($p<0.05$), hydatidiform mole group ($p<0.05$), and normal pregnancy group ($p<0.01$). There was no significant difference between any other combination of two groups.

Exploration of a Marker of Diagnostic Value

It was ascertained which one or ones of the three parameters (serum immunosuppressive effect, mononuclear cell reactivity to PHA, hCG) are useful for differentiating choriocarcinoma from invasive mole and/or for detecting metastasis. As a result, it was found that only the serum immunosuppressive effect significantly differed between the choriocarcinoma group and the invasive mole group ($p<0.10$) and also between the metastatic cases and the nonmetastatic cases ($p<0.05$) (Table 4).

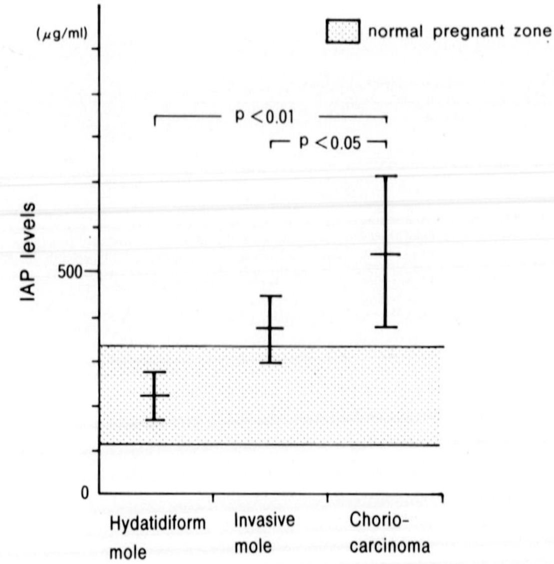

Figure 2. Serum immunosuppressive acidic protein (IAP) levels in patients with trophoblastic diseases.

Table 4. Comparison among various parameters and clinical status of trophoblastic diseases

Diseases		Parameter	
	Serum immuno-suppressive effect (% inhibition)	Mononuclear cell reactivity to PHA (cpm)	HCG (IU/liter)
Choriocarcinoma	49.4±27.5*	32,290±13,940	114,767±157,308
Invasive mole	23.7±28.6*	36,248±13,995	75,871±212,158
Metastasis (+)	52.7±26.9**	37,200±14,845	240,871±380,332
(−)	22.2±28.8**	31,514±13,661	162,294±394,329

* $p<0.10$, ** $p<0.05$.

Serum Immunosuppressive Effect and Prognosis

This parameter was studied to determine whether it is helpful for the prediction of prognosis. The product of this multiplication served as a prognostic score: amount of a drug prescribed during a course of treatment × number of courses. Consequently, the serum immunosuppressive effect determined before treatment correlated, though weakly, with the prognostic score (Figure 3).

Serum Immunosuppressive Effect and Clinical Effect

Changes in serum immunosuppressive effect, hCG level, and mononuclear cell reactivity to PHA were followed up during clinical course. In a representative case of clinical in-

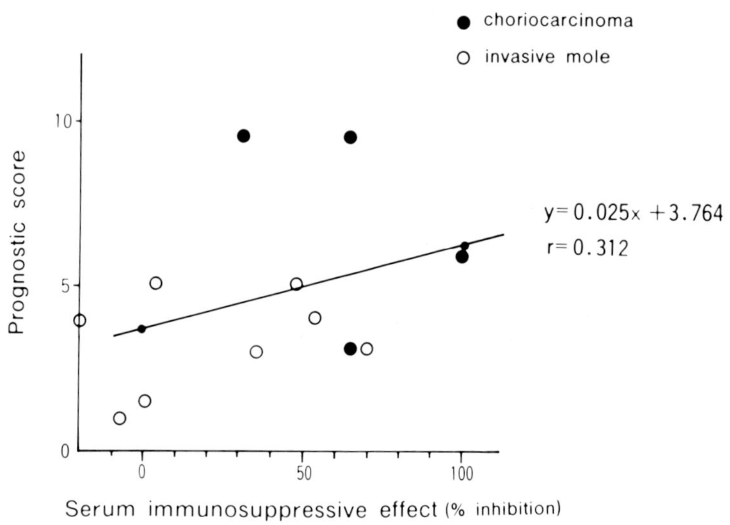

Figure 3. Serum immunosuppressive effect and prognosis.

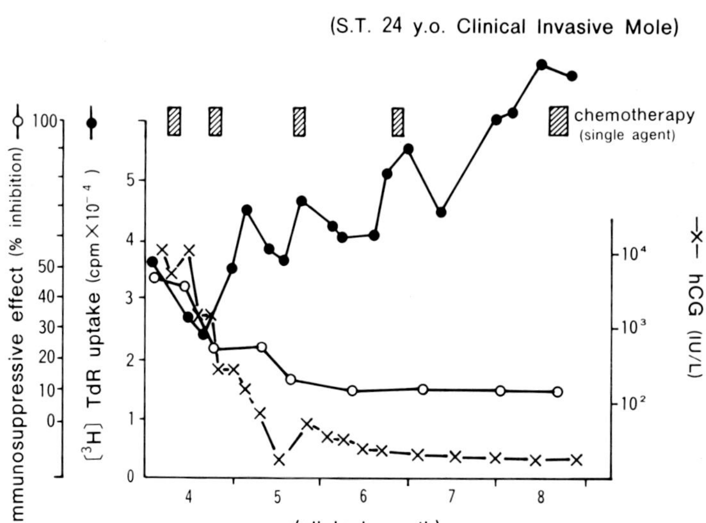

Figure 4. Changes in mononuclear cell reactivity to PHA, serum immunosuppressive effect, and hCG with clinical course.

vasive mole, the serum immunosuppressive effect was abated proportionally to the hCG level with advancing time. In contrast, the responsiveness of mononuclear cells to PHA stimulation was enhanced in inverse proportion to those two parameters (Figure 4). The cell-mediated immune capacity of this patient was improved as MAC (Methotrexate+Actinomycin D+Cyclophosphamide) therapy exerted a curative effect. In the case of clinical choriocarcinoma that was remitted by seven courses of chemotherapy, the serum immunosuppressive effect was reduced parallel with the hCG level. In this case, however,

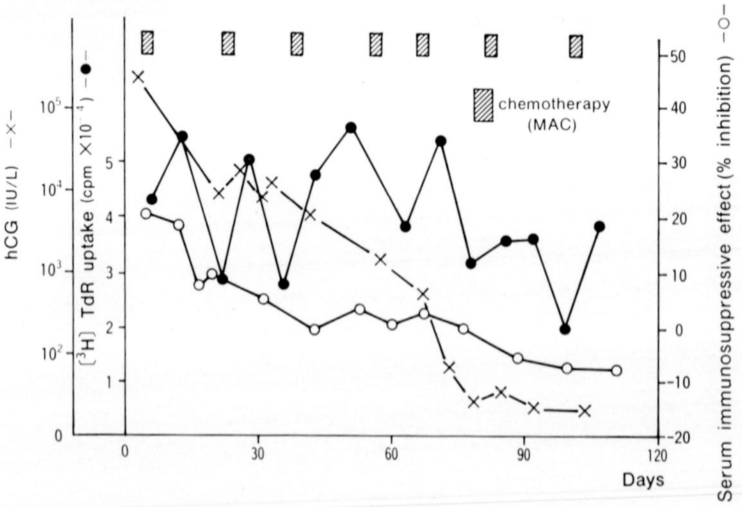

Figure 5. Changes in mononuclear cell reactivity to PHA, serum immunosuppressive effect, and hCG with clinical course (choriocarcinoma).

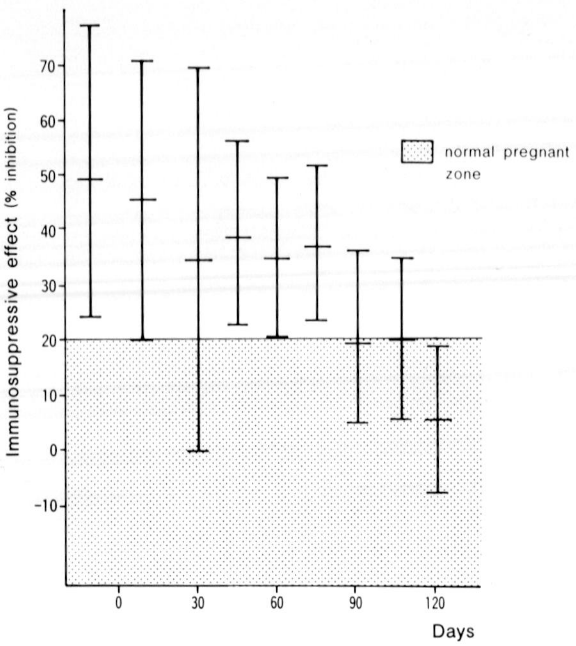

Figure 6. Changes in serum immunosuppressive effect after treatment (choriocarcinoma).

the PHA-reactivity of mononuclear cells was not augmented in spite of the therapeutic benefit (Figure 5).

The serum immunosuppressive effect was diminished in the choriocarcinoma group (Figure 6) and the invasive mole group (Figure 7) before treatment. In the former group, it came within the normal range 12 months after the start of treatment.

Serum Immunosuppressive Effect and Clinical Course of Hydatidiform Mole

The patients with hydatidiform mole were divided into two subgroups by the clinical

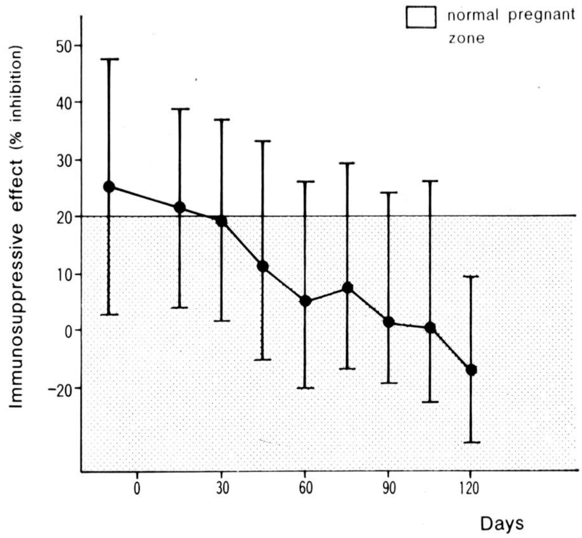

Figure 7. Changes in serum immunosuppressive effect after treatment (invasive mole).

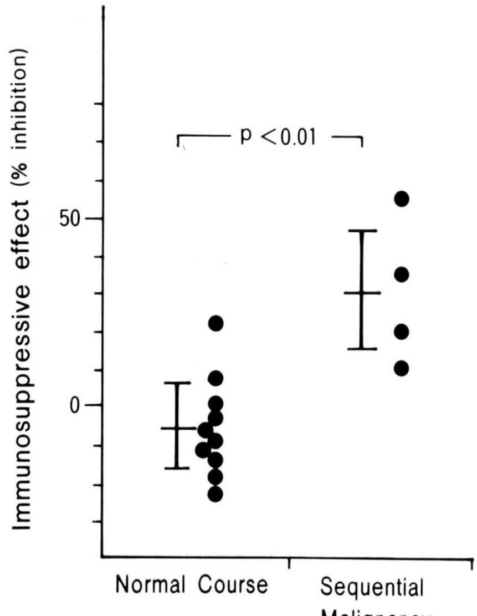

Figure 8. Comparison of serum immunosuppressive effect, ascertained at the stage of mole in utero, between normal course and sequential malignancy of hydatidiform mole.

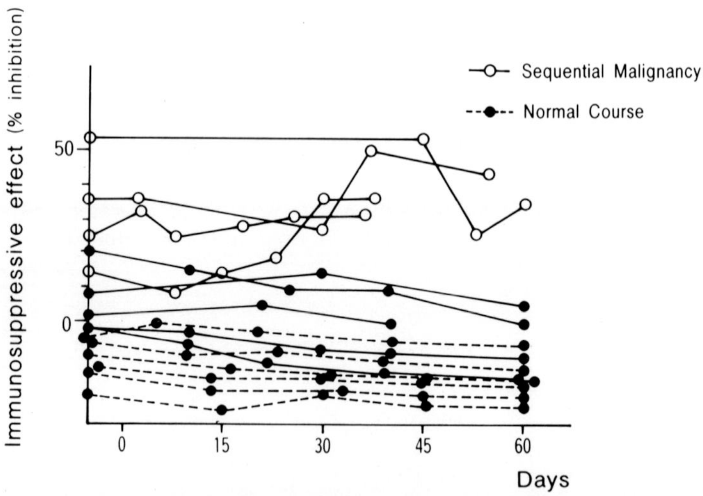

Figure 9. Changes in serum immunosuppressive effect in hydatidiform mole.

course after evacuation of the mole: sequential malignancy developed in one subgroup, and the postoperative course was uneventful in the other. In the sequential malignancy subgroup, the serum immunosuppressive effect was high in the state of mole in utero (Figure 8) and was maintained on a high level even after evacuation (Figure 9).

DISCUSSION

Trophoblastic disease is characterized as a lesion due to tumorous proliferation of chorionic villi that develop following fertilization. The lesion is recognized as a semiallograft by the host. It is presumed, therefore, that the immunologic response of the host is different from that of tumor-bearers in general. Among the three forms (hydatidiform mole, invasive mole, choriocarcinoma) of trophoblastic disease, invasive mole in itself belongs to mole and has to be clearly distinguished clinically from choriocarcinoma. There may also be an immunologic discrepancy between invasive mole and choriocarcinoma.

It has been reported that immunosuppressive factors exist in serum in tumor-bearers [12]. As trophoblastic diseases are related to pregnancy, various hormones are thought to act synergistically with those factors in serum in eliciting an immunosuppressive effect. In this connection, it was our belief that screening various immunological parameters would be useful for ascertainment of the pathological status of patients with trophoblastic diseases.

At first we studied the cellular immune capacity of our patients with trophoblastic diseases. The function of lymphocytes was investigated by the use of the most popular parameter, that is, mononuclear cell reactivity to PHA. This reactivity was determined by the whole blood microculture method, which we devised based on the procedure of Park and Good [8]. Briefly, these points characterize our method [19]: 1) No more than 0.05 mL of blood is required, and 2) it is not necessary to separate lymphocytes. Consequently our method is of high clinical value for determining the cell-mediated immune capacity, especially of T-cells, per unit of whole blood containing not only lymphocytes but also monocytes.

Comparison of mononuclear cell reactivity to PHA between the three forms of trophoblastic disease revealed that it was somewhat lowered in the choriocarcinoma group compared with the other two groups, as well as the normal pregnancy group. However, the differences involved were not statistically significant. This fact is construed as meaning that the lymphocyte function is maintained in choriocarcinoma, though it comes under the category of tumor. Accordingly, the ratio of clinically successful cases was high in the choriocarcinoma group.

This observation was not necessarily in agreement with the previous data. For instance, Takeuchi and Kanazawa [13] and Tomoda et al. [16] reported a significant decrease in lymphocyte reactivity to PHA in patients with choriocarcinoma. It must be pointed out, however, that they determined the reactivity per lymphocyte. Mano et al. [6], who employed a method similar to ours, found no significant decline in PHA-reactivity. Ho et al. [3], who used a procedure resembling that of Takeuchi and Kanazawa, reported that although the PHA-reactivity determined in the hydatidiform mole group after mole evacuation was significantly different from that in the malignant trophoblastic disease group, the value determined before evacuation was not. It was also reported that a decrease in PHA-reactivity was not observed in the mixed culture system using lymphocytes from patients as responder cells and those from other subjects as stimulator cells [4]. It can be surmised from the above that T-cell function is obviously not impaired in choriocarcinoma. However, we must pay due attention to the fact that the degree of impairment varies depending on the disease stages, as in uterine cancer [22].

On the other hand, consistent data have been published showing that the cell-mediated immune capacity determined in vivo by means of purified protein derivative (PPD) [11] or dinitrochlorobenzene (DNCB) [5] skin tests was decreased in choriocarcinoma. Those data thus suggest the presence of an in vivo mechanism that controls T-cell function. In this work, we studied serum immunosuppressive effect in patients with trophoblastic diseases by means of the whole blood microculture system using normal blood. The test serum added to this system was equivalent to 30% of the culture medium. According to this method, serum immunosuppressive effect was studied in three forms of trophoblastic disease, i.e., choriocarcinoma, invasive mole, and hydatidiform mole. Control subjects in the first trimester of gestation were used because they were considered more suitable than those in a later stage, particularly for comparison with patients with hydatidiform mole [18, 21]. The serum immunosuppressive effect was significantly greater in the choriocarcinoma group than in any of the other three groups, including the control group, but was not significantly different among these three groups. This increase in serum immunosuppressive effect was also reported by Moridaira [7]. We obtained similar comparative data concerning IAP.

It is intriguing that the serum immunosuppressive effect served as a useful parameter for differentiation between choriocarcinoma and invasive mole and between metastatic and nonmetastatic cases, whereas the other two parameters of hCG and mononuclear cell reactivity to mitogen failed to do so. In addition, that particular parameter furnished prognostic information. In fact, the stronger the pretreatment serum immunosuppressive effect was, the greater was the total dose required. Thus, it is conceivable that patients whose serum exerts a strong immunosuppressive effect are intractable. On the basis of his findings on DNCB skin tests, lymphocyte reactivity to PHA, and immunoglobulin levels in choriocarcinoma patients, Bagshawe [1] postulated that the prognosis of those patients whose immunocapacity is lowered might be unfavorable. However, in the present study it was not mononuclear cell reactivity to PHA, but serum immunosuppressive effect that correlated with prognosis.

The value of serum immunosuppressive effect as a marker of the efficacy of chemotherapy was estimated. It decreased nearly parallel with hCG in not only choriocarcinoma but invasive mole. Mononuclear cell reactivity to PHA was certainly increased with clinical course in cases of invasive mole that did not require lengthy treatment. However, in cases of choriocarcinoma requiring lengthy and intensive treatment, it was not increased even after remission of the condition, probably due to the side effect of the treatment. Therefore, this parameter was considered unsuitable for ascertaining curative effect. In sum, hCG was judged to be the best marker of the efficacy of treatment because of its high sensitivity and easy practicability.

The serum immunosuppressive effect ascertained in the hydatidiform mole group before evacuation was not significantly different from that in the invasive mole group, but classification of the cases of that group by the postoperative course produced interesting data. In the subgroup of the cases who suffered from sequential malignancy, the serum immunosuppressive effect in the state of mole in utero approximated that in the invasive mole group. On the other hand, in the subgroup of those whose postoperative course was uneventful, it was significantly lower. In the former subgroup, the serum immunosuppressive effect stayed on a high level even after evacuation. Although the number of cases we studied was too small to permit definitive conclusions, the above findings raise the possibility that the two subgroups were already pathologically different in the stage of mole in utero. Ho et al. [4] previously described this possibility, although another author [1] disagreed. Further studies are essential to clarify this controversial point.

In consequence, the present observations suggest that serum immunosuppressive effect is valuable for distinguishing choriocarcinoma from invasive mole, ascertaining the pathological condition of patients with trophoblastic disease, and predicting its prognosis and the development of malignancy sequential to hydatidiform mole.

Finally, consideration was given to immunosuppressive factors in patients with trophoblastic diseases, especially those with choriocarcinoma. As stated earlier in this report, choriocarcinoma is associated with a gravidic change, so that special attention is called to the role of hormones in immunosuppression. However, no correlation was reported between serum immunosuppressive effect and hCG [2, 9]. Mano et al. [6] did not recognize any correlation between immunosuppressive effect and cortisol or progesterone levels either. However, Ho et al. [3, 4] detected a serum factor specifically blocking MLR to the husbands' lymphocytes but not to the donor's lymphocytes in patients with choriocarchinoma, as in normal pregnant subjects [10]. That fact suggests the existence of a nonhormonal inhibitory factor in serum in choriocarcinoma as well as in normal pregnancy. On the other hand, the serum immunosuppressive effect had a weak correlation with the serum concentration of IAP [6, 20], a nonspecific immunosuppressive factor, in our patients with choriocarcinoma. In view of the fact that the IAP level is elevated in tumor-bearers as well, it may be reasonable to presume that there are factors common to choriocarcinoma and other carcinomas. In the meantime, Tsuji [17] detected a tumor cell-derived factor with strong immunosuppressive activity in the supernatant of choriocarcinoma cell culture.

From the foregoing it can be surmised that serum immunosuppressive effect in patients with trophoblastic diseases, especially those with choriocarcinoma, may be due to interinvolvement of gravidic factors, nonspecific factors as in tumor-bearers in general, and choriocarcinoma cell-derived factors.

REFERENCES

1. Bagshawe KD: Recent observations related to the chemotherapy and immunology of gestational choriocarcinoma. Advanced Cancer Res 18: 231, 1971.
2. Caidwell JL, Stites DP, Fudenberg HH: Human chorionic gonadotrophin: Effects of crude and purified preparations on lymphocyte responses to phytohemagglutinin and allogeneic stimulation. J Immunol 115: 1249, 1975.
3. Ho PC, Mak LW, Lawton JWM, Ma HK: Immunological parameters in gestational trophoblastic neoplasia. J Reprod Immunol 1: 307, 1980.
4. Ho PC, Wong LC, Lawton JWM, Ma HK: Mixed lymphocyte reaction in gestational trophoblastic disease: Presence of a specific plasma inhibitor of the response to paternal alloantigens. J Reprod Immunol 6: 105, 1984.
5. Kawasaki H: A study of cellular immunity in chorionic tumors and their prognosis. Acta Obstet Gynaecol Jpn 29: 1127, 1977.
6. Mano T, Goto S, Kaseki S, Tomoda U: Study on immuno-capacity in the patients with trophoblastic tumors. Acta Obstet Gynaecol Jpn 36: 303, 1984.
7. Moridaira H: Immuno-suppressive effect of sera in gynaecologic malignancies. Acta Obstet Gynaecol Jpn 31: 1320, 1979.
8. Park BH, Good RA: A new micromethod for evaluating lymphocyte responses to phytohemagglutinin. Quantitative analysis of the function of thymus-dependent cells. Proc Natl Acad Sci USA 69: 371, 1972.
9. Petrucco OM, Seamark RF, Holmes K, Forbes IJ, Symons RG: Changes in lymphocyte function during pregnancy. Br J Obstet Gynaecol 83: 245, 1976.
10. Rocklin RE, Kitzmiller JL, Carpenter CB, Garovoy MR, Pavid JR: Absence of an immunologic blocking factor from the serum of women with chronic abortus. N Engl J Med 22: 1209, 1976.
11. Sasaki T, Fujisaki S: Clinical studies on cell-mediated immunity in gestational trophoblastic disease: Nonspecific cellular immunocompetence in patients with hydatidiform mole and trophoblastic neoplasia. Microbiol Immunol 25: 387, 1981.
12. Silk M: Effect of plasma from patients with carcinoma on in vitro lymphocyte transformation. Cancer 20: 2088, 1967.
13. Takeuchi S, Kanazawa K: Changes of immunologic competence of lymphocytes evaluated by phytohemagglutinin (PHA) induced DNA synthesis related to pregnancy and gynecologic tumors. Acta Obstet Gynaecol Jpn 19: 59, 1972.
14. Takeuchi S: Criteria of trophoblastic diseases. Acta Obstet Gynaecol Jpn 36: 5, 1984.
15. Tamura K, Shibata Y, Matsuda Y, Ishida N: Isolation and characterization of immunosuppressive acidic protein from ascitic fluids of cancer patients. Cancer Res 41: 3244, 1981.
16. Tomoda Y, Fuma M, Saiki N, Ishizuka N, Akaza T: Immunologic studies in patients with trophoblastic neoplasia. Am J Obstet Gynecol 126: 661, 1976.
17. Tsuji Y: Immunosuppressive substance derived from choriocarcinoma. Acta Obstet Gynaecol Jpn 32: 627, 1980.
18. Ueda K, Nakamori H, Sako H, Umesaki N, Toyokawa M, Sugawa T: A role of maternal immune changes in the maintenance of conceptus and in the trigger of labor. Acta Obstet Gynaecol Jpn 29: 1151, 1977.
19. Ueda K, Toyokawa M, Nakamori H, Sako H, Umesaki N, Nakade J, Lee T, Sugawa T: Immunosuppressive effect of serum in patients with ovarian carcinoma. Obstet Gynecol 51: 225, 1978.
20. Umesaki N, Ooshika Y, Kawabata M, Sako H, Sugawa T: Immunosuppressive acidic protein levels in patients with gynecologic malignancy. J Jpn Soc Cancer Ther 17: 2056, 1982.
21. Walker FS, Freeman CB, Harris R: Lymphocyte reactivity in pregnancy. Br Med J 19: 469, 1972.
22. Yamagata S, Green GH: Cellular immune status of patients with pelvic cancer. Aust NZ J Obstet Gynaecol 16: 129, 1976.

6

Immunology in the Genesis of Hydatidiform Mole: Especially as Related to Immune Dependency of Trophoblastic Cell Growth in Vivo

Shoshichi Takeuchi

INTRODUCTION

Consensus now holds that complete hydatidiform mole (CHM) may arise from the ovum of androgenetic fertilization [6, 8, 10, 18, 29, 30]. This naturally prompts us to question why and how an androgenetic ovum leads to morphological formation of CHM. This presentation stresses the importance of the role of immunological mechanisms in morphogenesis of CHM arising from androgenetic ovum [21–24].

Morphologic features of CHM are 1) absence of an embryo, 2) formation of villous hydrops (molar vesicles) easily recognizable to the naked eye, 3) scantiness of blood vessels in the villous stroma, and 4) a variety of trophoblastic hyperplasia [21]. So far, chromosomal aberration has been classified either by anomaly of numbers and/or structures of chromosomes, but now abnormality of chromosomal origin such as androgenesis may well also be included in chromosomal aberration [23, 24]. It is very likely for the conceptus of androgenetic origin to give rise to early embryonal demise, probably in an ovular inner cell mass phase of embryonal development, due to its serious chromosomal anomaly. This may explain the absence of the embryo in CHM. But the trophoblastic cells may be considered to continue to survive the environment because they are very primitive in nature, as long as it is not hostile to them. Thus the trophoblasts could be considered to continue to function by their pinocytotic activity after the early demise of the embryo [1, 3]. Fetal angiogenesis is known to occur within the fifth week of gestation in normal conceptuses [3]. In androgenetic ovum, angiogenesis might be strongly disturbed because of early demise of the embryo by the fifth week of gestation. This may reasonably

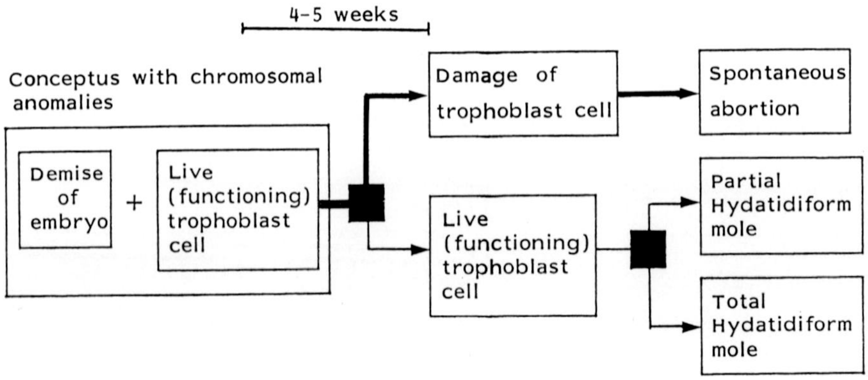

Figure 1. Nature's experimental model for elucidation of regulatory mechanism of trophoblast cell growth and damage.

explain the scantiness of fetal blood vessels in the villous stroma of CHM. Furthermore, the formation of villous hydrops could also be easily understood by the notion that water is liable to be retained in the villous stroma by the presence of the functioning trophoblasts in the absence of fetal circulation [3]. Regarding the morphogenesis of CHM, the most difficult question to be answered is why the trophoblasts continue to grow and survive, showing a variety of hyperplasia long enough to lead to formation of CHM in the absence of the embryo. It has been a common observation that conceptuses with chromosomal aberration such as triploidy, trisomy, and X monosomy may eventually result in spontaneous abortion (SpAb), with evidence of trophoblastic damage after demise of the embryo [1].

It is in this context that we examine nature's experimental model, as shown in Figure 1 [21–24]. The destiny of the conceptuses with chromosomal anomalies may be either SpAb with damaged trophoblasts or hydatidiform moles with a variety of trophoblastic hyperplasia after early demise of the embryo. Therefore, this model may provide a good experimental system for the study of the mechanism by which the growth of trophoblastic cells in vivo is regulated. Using this model, we propose that growth or damage of trophoblastic cells in vivo may be regulated by immunological mechanisms in which production of blocking antibodies (BAbs) evidenced by mixed leukocyte reaction (MLR) blocking assay may play a causal role in protecting the trophoblasts in vivo from immunological damage, the mechanisms of which are unknown [24].

Recently, immunogenic oncofetal antigens (OFA-I) were demonstrated to localize on the syncytiotrophoblast and found to produce an immunoglobulin (Ig) M antibody in the mother that may be cytotoxic to the trophoblast in the absence of BAbs [26, 27]. Therefore, this presentation will concentrate on the topic of immune dependency of trophoblastic cell growth in vivo.

METHODS

Viability of Fresh Trophoblastic Cells

This was evaluated by simultaneous staining with fluorescein diacetate-propidium iodide (FDA-PI), as reported by Jones and Sent (1985) [7].

Qualitative Determination of Trophoblast-Bound IgG and IgM in Various Early Pregnancies

Specimens were fixed in periodate-lysin-paraformaldehyde (PLP) fixative overnight and embedded in soft paraffin. After deparaffinization, indirect immunoperoxidase technique [13] was applied to the specimens. Rabbit Ig to human IgG (Dakopatts, Denmark) and rabbit Ig to human IgM (Dakopatts) were used as a first antibody, and horseradish peroxidase conjugated swine Ig to rabbit Ig (Dakopatts) as a second antibody.

Localization of OFA-I (GM_2) Antigens on Trophoblastic Cells

The indirect immunoperoxidase technique [13] used monoclonal antibody (mAb) produced by mouse hybridoma cell line 2B28a as a first antibody, and horseradish peroxidase conjugated rabbit Ig to mouse Ig (Dako).

An absorption test of anti-GM_2 antibody with trophoblastic plasma membrane vesicles [26] was done as follows. Anti-GM_2 antibody produced by the mouse hybridoma 2B28a was identified to be antibody to ganglioside M_2 (GM_2) [5]. Trophoblastic plasma membrane vesicles (TPMV) were obtained by the method described by Davies et al. (1985) [2] and tested whether anti-GM_2 antibody was absorbed by the TPMV. M-14 cell lines known to have GM_2 (OFA-I) antigens on their cell surface were used as target cells for detection of anti-GM_2 antibody using an immune adherence (IA) test.

MLR-Blocking Assay [20]

Mixed leukocyte culture reaction (MLR) was performed using the partner's lymphocytes treated with mitomycin as stimulator and the patient's lymphocytes as responder. Patient's sera or IgG fractions extracted from the patient's sera were added. Their blocking effect on one-way MLR was evaluated by the following formula:

$$\text{BE}(\%) = \left(1 - \frac{\text{mean cpm of culture in test serum}}{\text{mean cpm of culture in AB serum of IgG}}\right) \times 100.$$

RESULTS

Viability of Trophoblastic Cells Evaluated by FDA-PI Double Staining

Ten specimens of fresh trophoblastic tissues were obtained by dilatation and curettage from normal pregnancies in the first trimester (NP-1), hydatidiform moles, and SpAb, respectively. They were immediately stained with FDA-PI.

Most trophoblasts from SpAb were found to be damaged by propidium iodide-stained red color, whereas most trophoblasts from NP-1 and hydatidiform moles were found to be viable by evidence of fluorescein diacetate-stained green color [4].

Dynamics in Trophoblast-Bound IgG and IgM in Various Early Pregnancies

Trophoblasts in 204 cases of NP-1 obtained by artificial abortion done on basis of medical indications and those in 187 cases of SpAb were tested as to whether they were bound to IgG and/or IgM using indirect immunoperoxidase technique. We found that IgG but no IgM was always bound to cell surface of viable trophoblasts and IgM, but no IgG was often observed on the cell surface of damaged trophoblasts.

Then the positive rate of IgG or IgM bound to trophoblasts was analyzed and related to the duration of the trophoblasts staying in the uterus after early demise of the embryo in 57 cases of SpAb. These cases were selected by the criteria that the embryo was found and it was possible to evaluate the time of embryonal demise by crown-rump length

Table 1. Positive rate of immunoglobulin G and M bound to aborting trophoblasts related to the duration of persistence in the uterus after embryonal demise

Trophoblast-bound Ig	Duration after embryonal demise			Total
	4 wk	6 wk	8 wk	
IgG	46.2 (12/26)	15.0 (3/20)	9.1 (1/11)	28.1 (16/57)
IgM	34.6 (9/26)	60.0 (12/20)	63.6 (7/11)	45.6 (26/57)

Positive rate (%) $= \left(\frac{\text{No. of positive cases}}{\text{No. of examined cases}}\right) \times 100.$

(CRL) measurements and morphological features. The results are shown in Table 1. They indicate that IgG was being lost from the cell surface, and IgM was instead binding to the cell surface of the trophoblasts as the duration after demise of the embryo prolonged [25].

Localization of GM_2 (OFA-I) Antigens on Syncytiotrophoblasts

GM_2 antigens were found to localize on syncytiotrophoblasts in ten uteri of NP-1, and in five uteri of hydatidiform mole that were removed by surgery [25]. They were also observed to localize on syncytiotrophoblasts in ten delivered term placenta and ten placental tissues of SpAb obtained by dilatation and curettage [25].

The titer of anti-GM_2 antibody that is mouse monoclonal antibody to GM_2 was found to be significantly decreased by the absorption procedure with trophoblastic plasma membrane vesicles obtained from human term placenta, indicating the presence of GM_2 antigen on the trophoblastic membranes [26].

Kinetics in Production of BAbs (IgG) and Anti-GM_2 Antibodies (IgM) in Various States Related to Pregnancy

In first normal pregnancies, BAbs were observed to increase in amount to term as the gestational age advanced [9]. They were also found in total hydatidiform mole to continue to be produced in the absence of an embryo as evidenced by echogram. Their production, however, was not observed in 17 of 20 cases of unexplained habitual abortion and in 30 cases of SpAb [20]. Furthermore, vaccination with their partner's lymphocytes of the habitual aborters who lacked production of BAbs was found to cause production of BAbs. This might lead to BAbs production in new pregnancies, possibly allowing successful pregnancy [20].

Anti-GM_2 antibodies in sera were detected using an IA test with M-14 cell lines in more than 50% of first normal pregnancies, hydatidiform moles, and abortions, including incidental and habitual abortions [27].

DISCUSSION

The issue as to the immune dependency of trophoblastic cell growth in vivo has been a matter of speculation. The protective effect of IgG antibodies called blocking antibodies (BAbs), on trophoblastic growth and survival in vivo has been implicated, but the nature of BAbs has not yet been fully understood. Furthermore, any cogent evidence of immunological mechanism damaging trophoblasts in vivo has never been demonstrated, even in SpAbs with evidence of trophoblastic damage.

Keeping nature's experimental model (Figure 1) in mind, we have studied for nearly two decades the immunological difference between hydatidiform mole and SpAb in relation to NP-1. Prominent findings were that trophoblasts showing growth and survival as found in NP-1 and hydatidiform mole are always bound with IgG, but not with IgM on their cell surface [25], whereas those showing damage as found in SpAb are usually associated with binding with IgM and loss of IgG on their cell surface by indirect immunofluorescence [28] and indirect immunoperoxidase technique [25]. Also, in NP-1 and hydatidiform mole, the IgG BAbs evidenced by blocking effect of patients' sera on one-way MLR between partners are detected in most cases, whereas in SpAb these are not detected [9]. Another prominent finding was that IgM anti-OFA-I antibodies appeared in the sera from early first-pregnancies using IA assay with M-14 cell lines, but these antibodies were also detected in SpAb as well as in hydatidiform mole [27].

Thus the results obtained in our laboratory strongly suggested that humoral (antibody)-mediated immunity (HMI or AbMI) might play an important rôle in regulation of growth or damage of trophoblasts in vivo. However, the nature of anti-OFA-I antibodies (IgM) was not clarified before OFA-I antigens on M-14 cell membrane were chemically purified and identified as ganglioside GM_2 [5], and additionally mAb to GM_2 (OFA-I) was produced in the mouse [19].

As shown in this presentation, the presence of GM_2 (OFA-I) on the syncytiotrophoblasts of NP-1, hydatidiform mole, and SpAb was evidenced using indirect immunoperoxidase technique with mouse mAb to GM_2 [25] and absorption procedure of anti-GM_2 antibody with trophoblastic plasma membrane vesicles [26]. Therefore, the reason why antibody to OFA-I antigens was often detected by IA assay with M-14 cells in the sera from normal pregnant women, moral patients, and aborting women might be easily explained. Furthermore, we found that in the sera from the nonpregnant unexplained habitual aborters, anti-OFA-I antibodies were detected [17]. From these findings, it is tempting to speculate that IgM bound to damaged trophoblast must be anti-GM_2 (OFA-I) antibody.

On the other hand, it was confirmed in our laboratory that BAbs may include at least antibodies against HLA-D/DR antigens presented on the partner's lymphocytes [9, 11, 15]. In addition, other investigators have reported that BAbs may include the anti-Fc-receptor blocking antibody [14], the antiidiotypic antibody to maternal lymphocytes [16], and/or the anti-TLX antibody [12]. Whatever the true nature of BAbs, we believe that they may be an indispensable protective factor for survival of trophoblasts in vivo, based on the results obtained in our laboratory.

Immunological data obtained in our laboratory, summarized in Table 2, are related to the prominent growth pattern of trophoblastic cells observed morphologically in various early pregnancies. We thus interestingly noted the fact that viable trophoblasts found in normal pregnancies and hydatidiform moles are associated with coexistence of IgG-BAbs and IgM-anti-GM_2 antibodies in sera and binding of only IgG with their cells; however, damaged trophoblasts observed in SpAb and habitual abortion are associated with the presence of IgM-anti-GM_2 antibodies in the absence of IgG-BAbs in sera and binding of only IgM with their cell surface. Therefore it may be suggested, as depicted in Figure 2, that IgM-anti-GM_2 antibody may be cytotoxic to trophoblasts in vivo in the presence of complement and IgG antibodies may protect trophoblasts from their damage by preventing binding of cytotoxic IgM with trophoblasts. However, in the absence of BAbs, cytotoxic IgM may bind to trophoblasts after losing IgG binding to them, thus eventually resulting in their damage. It is therefore tempting to speculate, in an analogy to the TLX hypothesis [12], that trophoblastic cells may have at least two alloantigens: one is trophoblast

Table 2. Immunological data related to the prominent growth pattern of trophoblastic cells in various pregnancies

Pregnancy	Prominent growth pattern of trophoblasts	Alloantigens on trophoblasts		Trophoblast-bound immunoglobulin		Antibodies in sera	
		TA-G (?)	TA-M (GM2)	IgG	IgM	BAbs (IgG)	GM2Abs (IgM)
Normal	Viable, two layer	+	+	+	−	+	+
Hydatidiform mole	Viable, a variety of hyperplasia	+	+	+	−	+∼⧺	+
Spontaneous abortion	Damaged	+	+	−	−∼+	−	+
Habitual abortion	Damaged	−∼+	+	−	+	−	+

+=present; −=absent; ⧺=strongly present; ∼= or.

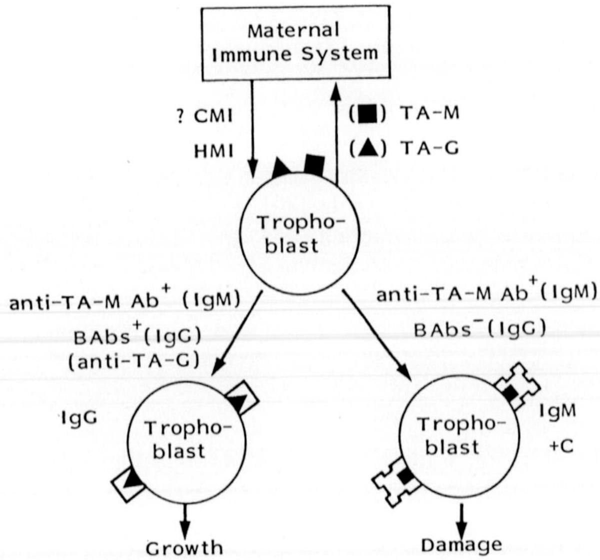

Figure 2. Immune dependency of trophoblastic cell growth in vivo. ■ TA-M=OFA-I (GM_2); ▲ TA-G=? HLA-D/DR linked TLX-like substance; ⌘ anti-TA-M Ab: anti-OFA-I (GM_2) antibody (IgM); ◸ BAbs (blocking antibodies)=anti-TA-G Ab (Anti-TA-G antibody) (IgG); CMI=cell-mediated immunity; HMI=humoral-mediated immunity; +=production (or the presence); −=no production (or the absence).

antigen (TA) to produce IgG-BAb (TA-G), and the other is TA to produce IgM (TA-M) that is anti-GM_2 antibody (TA-M = GM_2).

CONCLUSION

Survival or damage of trophoblasts may be regulated by protective IgG-BAbs and cytotoxic IgM-GM_2 antibody produced to two alloantigens on them—TA-G and TA-M antigens. The nature of the TA-G antigens is considered HLA D/DR-linked-TLX-like, but remains unknown; and the nature of the TA-M antigens is identified as GM_2. Growth and survival of trophoblasts may be sustained by the presence of BAbs, even in coexistence with cytotoxic

IgM antibody, whereas damage of trophoblasts may be achieved by cytotoxic IgM antibody in the absence of BAbs.

In development of androgenetic ova, early demise of embryos occurs, probably in the ovular phase of their development, thus leading to 1) the absence of the embryo, and to 2) scantiness of blood vessels in villous stroma. Alloantigens on trophoblasts may strongly be expressed because of paternal origin of all chromosomes. This is followed by the fact that trophoblasts continue to grow and survive by continuing production of IgG BAbs, thus showing 3) a variety of trophoblastic hyperplasia, leading to 4) formation of molar vesicles by the pinocytotic activity of trophoblasts in the absence of embryonal circulation.

Morphogenesis of CHM from androgenetic ova thus may be described by in terms of immunology, which explains immune dependency of trophoblastic growth in vivo.

REFERENCES

1. Car DH: Chromosomes and abortion. In Harris H, Hirshorn K (eds): Advances in Human Genetics. Plenum, New York, 1971, p. 201.
2. Davies M, Parry JE, Sutcliffe RG: Examination of different preparations of human placental plasma membrane for the binding of insulin, transferrin and immunoglobulins. J Reprod Fertil 63: 315, 1981.
3. Hertig AT: Hydatidiform mole and chorionepithelioma. In Meigo JV, Sturgis SH (eds): Progress in Gynecology, Vol 2. 1950, p. 372.
4. Honma S, Takeuchi S: Determination of cell viability of trophoblasts in vivo by simultaneous staining with fluorescein diacetate-propidium iodate. (to be published).
5. Irie RF, Tai T, Morton DL: Antibodies to tumor-associated gangliosides (GM_2 and GD_2); Potential for suppression of melanoma recurrence. In Basic Mechanism and Clinical Treatment of Tumor Metastasis. 1985, p. 371.
6. Jacobs PA, Wilson C, Sprenkle J, et al.: Mechanism of origin of complete hydatidiform moles. Nature 286: 714, 1980.
7. Jones KH, Sent JA: An improved method to determine cell viability by simultaneous staining with fluorescein diacetate-propidium iodide. J Histochem Cytochem 33: 77, 1985.
8. Kajii T, Ohama K: Androgenetic origin of hydatidiform mole. Nature 268: 633, 1980.
9. Kajino T, Kanazawa K, Takeuchi S: Blocking effects of maternal serum-IgG and placental eluate-IgG on materno-fetal mixed lymphocyte reaction and their individual specificity. Am J Reprod Immunol 4: 27, 1983.
10. Lawler D, Povey T, Fisher A, Pickthall J: Genetic studies on hydatidiform mole; II. The origin of complete mole. Ann Hum Genet 46: 232, 1982.
11. Maruhashi T, Takakuwa T, Kajino T, et al.: Characterization and detection of blocking antibodies in early pregnant sera. Am J Reprod Immunol 5: 99, 1984.
12. McIntyre JA, Faulk WP: Allotypic trophoblast-lymphocyte cross-reactive (TLX) cell surface antigens. Hum Immunol 1982: 4, 1982.
13. Nakane P, Pierce GB: Enzyme-labeled antibodies for the light and electron microscopic localization of tissue antigens. J Cell Biol 33: 307, 1967.
14. Power DA, Catto GRD, Mason RJ, MacLeod AM, Stewart GM, Stewart KN, Shewan WG: The fetus as an allograft; Evidence for protective antibodies to HLA-linked paternal antigens. Lancet 2: 701, 1983.
15. Rocklin RE, Kitzmiller JL, Garvoy MR: Maternal-fetal relation; II. Further characterization of an immunologic blocking factor that develops during pregnancy. Clin Immunol Immunopathol 22: 305, 1982.
16. Suciu-Foca N, Reed E, Rohowsky C, Kung P, King DW: Antiidiotypic antibodies to anti-HLA receptors induced by pregnancy. Proc Natl Acad Sci USA 80: 830, 1983.
17. Suzuki T, Takakuwa K, Takuechi S: The presence of anti-OFA-I (GM_2) antibody evidenced by immune adherence test with M-14 target cells in the sera from the habitual aborters with evidence of the absence of seral blocking antibody. (to be published).
18. Szulman AE, Surti U: Complete and partial moles; cytogenetic and morphological aspects. In Pattillo RA, Hussa RO (eds): Human Trophoblast Neoplasms. Plenum, New York, 1984, p. 136.
19. Tai T, Paulson JC, Cahan LD, Irie RF: Ganglioside GM_2 as a human tumor antigen (OFA-I-I). Proc Natl Acad Sci 80: 5392, 1983.
20. Takakuwa K, Kanazawa K, Takeuchi S: Production of blocking antibodies by vaccination in unexplained recurrent aborters and their role for successful pregnancy. Am J Reprod Immunol Microbiol 10: 1986.

21. Takeuchi S, Hando T, Honda T, et al.: The nature of "Trophoblastic Tumours"; Immunological and pathological approach. J Asian Fed Obstet Gynecol 2: 218, 1971.
22. Takeuchi S: Immunology of spontaneous abortion and hydatidiform mole. Am J Reprod Immunol 1: 23, 1980.
23. Takeuchi S: Immunology of growth and demise of embryo-trophoblast unit indicated by comparative study between abortion and hydatidiform mole—A nature's experiment system. In Ray PK (ed): Immunobiology of Transplantation, Cancer and Pregnancy. Pergamon, Elmsford, New York, 1983, p. 305.
24. Takeuchi S: Immunology in genesis of partial and total hydatidiform mole. In Pattillo RA, Houssa RO (eds): Human Trophoblast Neoplasms. Plenum, New York, 1984, p. 81.
25. Takeuchi S, Obata N, Sasagawa M: Dynamics of trophoblast-bound IgG and IgM after the early demise of the embryo. (to be published).
26. Takeuchi S, Suzuki T, Sasagawa M: The localization of OFA-I (GM_2) antigens on trophoblastic cell membranes producing IgM antibody. (to be published).
27. Takeuchi Y: The clinical significance of OFA-I in immunological rejection mechanism to trophoblasts (in Japanese). Acta Obstet Gynecol Jpn 37: 1893, 1985.
28. Tokunaga A: Studies of humoral immunological response on the aborted trophoblasts (in Japanese). Acta Obstet Gynecol Jpn 33: 2125, 1981.
29. Wake N, Takagi N, Sasaki M: Androgenesis as a cause of hydatidiform mole. J Natl Cancer Inst 60: 51, 1978.
30. Yamashita K, Wake N, et al.: A further HLA study of hydatidiform moles. Gynecol Oncol 11: 238, 1981.

7

Gestational Trophoblast Neoplasms: Immunity of Mother and Child

Roland A. Pattillo

INTRODUCTION

The detection of choriocarcinoma in the placenta of a patient with gestational choriocarcinoma has been reported only several times in the world literature [1–9]. This may be largely due to the fact that the placenta is no longer available for study when the diagnosis of choriocarcinoma is made in the mother. The time of transformation from normal trophoblast to choriocarcinoma cannot be determined for certain; however, the fact that several cases have been reported in which the malignancy existed within the placenta indicates that this malignant transformation may take place during the gestational period. Malignant transformation in trophoblast cells retained after expulsion of the placenta cannot be excluded.

Rarely, gestational choriocarcinoma may be transmitted transplacentally to the fetus, resulting in the birth of a child with choriocarcinoma or one that manifests the malignancy at a later date. Characteristically, the child of a gestational choriocarcinoma is normal and does not give evidence of disease. This study will report the results of a study of mothers with choriocarcinoma and the manifestation of immunological sensitivity to that malignancy by the mother and the child of the respective pregnancy. Eighteen mothers were studied using a cytotoxicity assay (modified Helstrom assay) that identifies immunological recognition of choriocarcinoma cells by lymphocytes sensitized to this malignancy in the mother and in the offspring of that pregnancy in the postnatal period. All children studied showed immunological recognition of choriocarcinoma target cells in vitro and displayed no blocking of cytotoxicity. All mothers showed immunological recognition, cytotoxicity, and blocking of cytotoxicity only when choriocarcinoma was present as evidenced by positive human chorionic gonadotropin (hCG) levels. One infant in the study died with metastatic choriocarcinoma. Children of these choriocarcinoma mothers have been studied at various points corresponding to key points in maturation of immunological competence as relates to postnatal development of the immune system. The data represents only a preliminary report, as limited opportunities are available for obtaining adequate blood samples from infants and children of choriocarcinoma mothers. Such an attempt to suggest a structural framework for the development of immunological reactivity to neoplastic trophoblast antigens will be understandably limited in potentital. Nonetheless, the availability of the trophoblast model in vitro permits the initial opportunity to elucidate previously unknown dimensions.

MATERIALS AND METHODS

Blocking factor assays at this center have recently been added to hCG monitoring of trophoblast disease patients because of an approximate 10% incidence of recurrent disease after chemotherapy. Blocking factor is a new test for agents in the patient's serum that prevent the host from reacting against the tumor. It may be tumor antigen, tumor antibody, or antigen antibody complex.

The blocking factor assay consists of incubation of choriocarcinoma target cells with the patient's lymphocytes and controls. The choriocarcinoma cells are grown without lymphocytes; with normal control lymphocytes (which do not antigenically recognize the tumor cells, and therefore do not adhere); and with the patient's lymphocytes. The patient's lymphocytes are specifically sensitized to the tumor, recognize it, and cytotoxically destroy it unless the patient's serum, which contains the blocking factor and prevents the lymphocytes from adhering and destroying the tumor, is added. The endpoint of the assay is terminal tritiated thymidine uptake of target tumor cells not destroyed by the cytotoxic lymphocytes. The blocking index is calculated by the difference of cytotoxicity in the presence and absence of the patient's serum containing the blocking factor. The choriocarcinoma cells were derived from five different patients.

The blocking factor calculation (Table 1) was performed as previously described [10, 11]. The choriocarcinoma cells were grown in tissue culture flasks and transferred to Lab Tek chambers for the assay. In the absence and in the presence of the patient's serum, 1,000 target choriocarcinoma cells were incubated with 100,000 lymphocytes from the patient. If blocking was present, cytotoxic destruction of choriocarcinoma cells would be blocked when the patient's serum was added to the incubation. The blocking index could be calculated as the difference between cytotoxicity in the absence and in the presence of the patient's serum. A pulse procedure with tritiated thymidine was used to

Table 1. Blocking factor assay

Control	Experiment
10^3 target cells	10^3 target cells
10^5 patient's lymphocytes with patient's serum	10^5 patient's lymphocytes without patient's serum
24-hr incubation	24-hr incubation
2-hr thymidine pulse	2-hr thymidine pulse

Blocking index = lymphocyte killing with patient's serum − lymphocyte killing without patient's serum.

detect the remaining undestroyed tumor cells after incubation. Target cells (10^3 cells/well) were incubated in eight well Lab Tek chambers at 37°C in an atmosphere of 5% CO_2 in air. After 24 hours incubation, the medium was removed and replaced with fresh 3520 medium (30% Geys balanced salt solution, 50% Waymouth medium, 20% fetal calf serum; Grand Island Biologic, Grand Island, New York) containing 10^5 lymphocytes or 3520 medium with 20% patient's serum containing 10^5 lymphocytes. After incubation for 24 hours, the chambers were washed four times with balanced salt solution (BSS) to remove the lymphocytes. The remaining target cells were incubated for 2 hours in 3520 medium with ^3H thymidine (10 μCi/ml, 5 to 30 Ci/mmol). The pulse medium was removed, and the cells were washed twice with BSS containing excess unlabeled thymidine, and frozen. After thawing, the amount of radioactivity incorporated into acid-precipitable material was determined. Determinations were made in triplicate. Values were expressed as percentage of radioactivity incorporated by target cells incubated in the absence of lymphocytes. Cytotoxicity of patient's lymphocytes was assessed by comparing values obtained from incubations of patient lymphocytes versus normal donor lymphocytes incubated with target in the same assay. Blocking of cytotoxicity was assessed by comparing values obtained from incubation of patient lymphocytes in fetal calf serum-containing medium versus autologous serum containing medium with target cells in the assay. Significance was assessed by student's T-test, with $p<0.05$ considered significant.

RESULTS

As described in the Materials and Methods section, the modified Helstrom assay has been used as a cytotoxicity and blocking factor assay and has been shown to correlate with the sensitive tumor marker hCG. Table 2 is a representative series of assays in a patient studied over a prolonged longitudinal period. The patient demonstrated positive cytotoxity in approximately 75% of the tests in which she was studied. Conditions that may produce failed cytotoxicity include poor growth of target cells, poor dispersion of sensitized lymphocytes, mechanical factors, and others.

Table 3 shows a series of trophoblast disease mothers, all of whom displayed cytotoxicity in the assay system. Patient CoCl (Table 4) is an example of a patient who demonstrated recognition, cytotoxicity, and blocking during the time when progressive choriocarcinoma growth was present. Upon surgical and chemotherapeutic resolution of tumor, this patient continued to show recognition and cytotoxicity, but demonstrated disappearance of blocking of cytotoxicity.

Table 5 shows the results for patient LaDe of multiple target cell choriocarcinoma system studies, all of which showed recognition of choriocarcinoma target cells by the patient's sensitized lymphocytes. These assays confirm the Helstrom phenomena that lymphocytes from patients bearing similar histologic-type tumor sensitize the lymphocytes to this tumor-associated antigen, which is cross-reactive with other tumors of the same histologic type. Control assays with other malignant target cells including cervix, breasts, and ovarian cancer target cells are uniformly negative for cross-reactivity.

Patients LuLu and DeWe, whose results are shown in Tables 6 and 7, showed recognition and cytoxicity. However, they were persistently blocked, with positive hCG titers. These patients are known to have metastatic choriocarcinoma.

Results for patient JAr, a choriocarcinoma mother and her child following the gestation, are shown in Table 8. This mother is in continuous remission from her gestational

Table 2. Blocking factor assay—Patient LiWi

JAr cells mo/yr	Control lymphocytes	Patient lymphocytes	Patient lymphocytes with autologous serum	Recognition	Blocking
2/81	112.1*± 7.6†	20.2± 6.5	100.4±15.7	+‡	+§
2/81	123.1 ±24.5	43.9± 5.0	93.7±23.8	+	+
3/81	132.0 ± 9.5	18.9±12.9	79.2± 2.2	+	+
12/81	85.6 ±18.1	47.1± 7.5	71.2±18.4	+	—
1/82	102.1 ± 8.6	34.0± 3.2	64.9±20.7	+	+
2/82	93.0 ±12.5	90.2±27.6	160.4±23.1	—‖	ND¶
2/82	111.4 ±10.1	49.3±13.0	114.7±29.9	+	+
4/82	87.1 ±20.5	88.2±11.7	132.3±73.5	—	ND
4/82	87.0 ±12.9	77.7± 5.5	142.5±16.6	—	ND
4/82	88.9 ±13.7	41.2± 9.7	125.8±11.5	+	+
4/82	134.0 ±17.7	19.7± 4.5	130.0±29.7	+	+
5/82	105.9 ±11.7	64.4± 0.03	102.1±23.8	+	—
5/82	105.4 ±21.9	30.6±24.7	59.8± 3.5	+	—
5/82	106.5 ±34.4	81.9±14.1	107.6±13.4	—	ND
6/82	135.8 ±10.7	72.8± 8.7	106.6±15.8	+	+
6/82	126.0 ±20.7	64.4± 6.1	138.0±34.2	+	+
4/83	104.9 ±14.6	40.0±18.1	97.0±15.0	+	+
5/83	110.3 ±10.5	38.6±19.8	103.9±23.6	+	+

* Percent lymphocytes.
† Mean±SE.
‡ Differs significantly ($p \leq 0.05$) from target cells incubated with control lymphocytes.
§ Differs significantly ($p \leq 0.05$) from target cells incubated with patient lymphocytes.
‖ Not significantly different.
¶ Not determined.
+=present; —=absent.

Table 3. Blocking factor assay

Patient	Recognition and blocking of cytotoxicity
CoCl	+
LaDe	+
LiLi	+
ElFa	+
JAr	+
BarN	+
DoSmi	+
MaBr	+
DiBl	+
CaPl	+
LuLu	+
DeWe	+
LiWi	+
DoMi	+
SEb	+
KaOl	+
MaGu	+
KaKu	+
Total	18

+=present.

Table 4. Blocking factor assay—Patient CoCl

Omega-Z cells mo/yr	Control lymphocytes	Patient lymphocytes	Patient lymphocytes with autologous serum	Recognition	Blocking
1/81	109.3*±22.3†	13.1±7.8	115.1±17.5	+‡	+§
2/81	105.9 ± 6.6	11.1±7.9	18.8±11.5	+	–

* Percent lymphocytes.
† Mean±SE.
‡ Differs significantly ($p \leqq 0.05$) from target cells incubated with control lymphocytes.
§ Differs significantly ($p \leqq 0.05$) from target cells incubated with patient lymphocytes.

Table 5. Blocking factor assay—Patient LaDe

JAr cells mo/yr	Control lymphocytes	Patient lymphocytes	Patient lymphocytes with autologous serum	Recognition	Blocking
1/81	108.2*± 9.6†	54.1± 3.7	128.8±17.9	+‡	+§
2/81	82.4 ± 9.1	23.4± 4.1	78.6±20.1	+	+
2/81	123.1 ±24.5	18.9±13.9	18.9± 3.4	+	–
3/81	133.3 ± 5.5	11.3± 1.7	28.5± 4.1	+	+
2/83	141.7 ±12.1	34.3± 6.7	39.1±13.0	+	–
BeWo cells					
3/81	139.8 ±17.1	4.4± 0.8	5.5± 1.1	+	–
4/81	96.9 ±18.9	9.4± 1.0	13.7± 4.0	+	–
ElFa cells					
3/81	148.0 ±14.2	15.7± 2.6	20.1± 4.3	+	–
4/81	105.1 ±17.2	0.3± 6.5	72.1± 4.9	+	+
Omega-Z cells					
1/81	109.8 ±22.3	28.5±27.7	94.3±35.6	+	–
3/81	147.2 ±12.8	15.6± 5.2	16.6±13.8	+	–

* Percent lymphocytes.
† Mean±SE.
‡ Differs significantly ($p \leqq 0.05$) from target cells incubated with control lymphocytes.
§ Differs significantly ($p \leqq 0.05$) from target cells incubated with patient lymphocytes.

Table 6. Blocking factor assay—Patient LuLu

JAr cells mo/yr	Control lymphocytes	Patient lymphocytes	Patient lymphocytes with autologous serum	Recognition	Blocking
2/83	113.4*±15.2†	43.4± 5.4	96.0±23.2	+‡	+§

* Percent lymphocytes.
† Mean±SE.
‡ Differs significantly ($p \leqq 0.05$) from target cells incubated with control lymphocytes.
§ Differs significantly ($p \leqq 0.05$) from target cells incubated with patient lymphocytes.

Table 7. Blocking factor assay—Patient DeWe

JAr cells mo/yr	Control lymphocytes	Patient lymphocytes	Patient lymphocytes with autologous serum	Recognition	Blocking
6/82	126.0*±20.7†	63.9±11.4	134.2±18.7	+‡	+§
6/82	93.4 ±10.9	56.7± 4.1	102.8±14.0	+	+

* Percent lymphocytes.
† Mean±SE.
‡ Differs significantly ($p \leq 0.05$) from target cells incubated with control lymphocytes.
§ Differs significantly ($p \leq 0.05$) from target cells incubated with patient lymphocytes.

Table 8. Blocking factor assay—Choriocarcinoma patient (JAr) and child

JAr choriocarcinoma cells mo/yr	Control lymphocytes	Patient lymphocytes	Patient lymphocytes with autologous serum	Recognition	Blocking
Mother					
6/80	100.5± 4.6	41.8±15.9	35.4±17.0	+	—
12/81	130.0± 0.1	67.3± 1.9	75.0± 9.6	+	—
6/82	93.4±10.9	49.7± 8.0	79.1±18.7	+	—
12/83	113.7±15.2	16.1± 5.3	8.5± 4.3	+	—
Child					
6/80	100.5± 4.6	53.9±21.6	44.9±19.0	+	—
12/81	130.0± 0.1	44.2±13.4	73.0±11.5	+	—
12/83	113.7±15.2	7.3± 0.4	11.9± 2.4	+	—

+=present; —=absent.

Table 9. Blocking factor assay—Choriocarcinoma patient (MaDa) and male child, age 5 months

JAr choriocarcinoma cells mo/yr	Control lymphocytes	Patient lymphocytes	Patient lymphocytes with autologous serum	Recognition	Blocking
Mother					
12/83	92.1±9.7	51.3±4.5	65.3±21.4	+	—
Child					
Died of metastatic choriocarcinoma					

+=present; —=absent.

choriocarcinoma and, as indicated in Table 8, continues to show recognition and cytotoxicity against her own choriocarcinoma cells and absence of blocking factor activity. The child of that choriocarcinoma pregnancy, likewise shown in Table 8, similarly shows recognition and cytotoxicity against the placental choriocarcinoma of the respective gestation and shows no blocking activity.

In contrast to the above case of a healthy child free of choriocarcinoma but demonstrating immunologic memory of this event during pregnancy, Table 9 shows a child who died at age 5 months from metastatic choriocarcinoma. Although the mother, patient MaDa, remained healthy without clinical evidence of choriocarcinoma, her lymphocytes showed recognition and cytotoxicity without blocking factor activity, indicating sensitization by this choriocarcinoma tumor-associated antigen.

The following studies of mothers and children show assays conducted at periodic points in the postnatal development of the children of these pregnancies. Table 10 shows the

Table 10. Blocking factor assay—Choriocarcinoma patient (CoCl) and female child, age 3 years

JAr choriocarcinoma cells mo/yr	Control lymphocytes	Patient lymphocytes	Patient lymphocytes with autologous serum	Recognition	Blocking
Mother					
12/83	113.7*±15.2†	19.9±3.2	16.2±2.4	+‡	−§
Child					
12/83				+	−

* Percent lymphocytes.
† Mean±SE.
‡ Differs significantly ($p \leq 0.05$) from target cells incubated with control lymphocytes.
§ Differs significantly ($p \leq 0.05$) from target cells incubated with patient lymphocytes.
+=present; −=absent.

Table 11. Blocking factor assay—Choriocarcinoma patient (LiLi) and female child, age 4 years

JAr choriocarcinoma cells mo/yr	Control lymphocytes	Patient lymphocytes	Patient lymphocytes with autologous serum	Recognition	Blocking
Mother					
10/80	154.7±26.5	7.3± 3.6	50.7±10.3	+	+
2/81	82.4± 9.1	45.7±14.8	57.1±29.3	+	−
Child					
12/83	113.7±15.2	10.4± 0.4	ND ND	+	ND

ND=not determined; +=present; −=absent.

Table 12. Blocking factor assay—Choriocarcinoma patient (DiBi) and female child, age 5 years

JAr choriocarcinoma cells mo/yr	Control lymphocytes	Patient lymphocytes	Patient lymphocytes with autologous serum	Recognition	Blocking
Mother					
1/84	94.4±11.1	38.6±15.9	64.7±18.4	+	−
Child					
1/84	94.4±11.1	40.3±12.6	50.1± 5.5	+	−

+=present; −=absent.

results for patient CoCl and her child, who was studied at 3 years of age. At that time the child showed recognition and cytotoxicity of JAr choriocarcinoma cells in the same fashion as her mother, who was in complete remission.

The results for patient LiLi, along with those of her child at 4 years of age, are shown in Table 11. At that time both mother and child showed recognition and cytotoxicity, without blocking in the mother after resolution of her choriocarcinoma in February 1981.

Patient DiBi was studied together with her child at 5 years of age. Recognition and cytotoxicity were shown in both mother and child (Table 12).

To determine whether male or female offspring would produce differences in cytotoxicity, Tables 13 and 14 show, respectively, a female and male child of postgestational choriocarcinoma in which the mother died of metastatic disease. Both the male and female child are living free of disease, and show recognition and cytotoxicity to the choriocarcinoma antigens of the mother.

Previous reports have suggested a higher frequency of choriocarcinoma in blood type

Table 13. Blocking factor assay—Z in female child, age >10 years

Mother: Z-chorio-carcinoma cells mo/yr	Control lymphocytes	Patient lymphocytes	Patient lym-phocytes with autologous serum	Recognition	Blocking
Child 3/82	93.6±15.0	57.6± 9.9	26.6±12.8	+	–

+=present; –=absent.

Table 14. Blocking factor assay—BeWo in male child, age >10 years

Mother: BeWo chorio-carcinoma mo/yr	Control lymphocytes	Patient lymphocytes	Phocytes with autologous serum	Recognition	Blocking
Child 1/80	129.8±29.8	31.5±5.2	115.7±73.6	+	–

+=present; –=absent.

Table 15. Blocking factor assay—Choriocarcinoma patient (JAr) and male child, age >10 years

BeWo chorio-carcinoma cells mo/yr	Control lymphocytes	Patient lymphocytes	Patient lym-phocytes with autologous serum	Recognition	Blocking
Mother 12/83	76.6±4.6	13.0±4.1	17.4±2.3	+	–
Child 12/83	76.6±4.6	12.1±3.1	28.3±8.9	+	–

+=present; –=absent.

A mothers. It was of interest to determine if the child of such a pregnancy was different in any way from other postgestational choriocarcinoma infants. Table 15 shows no difference in the assay system of the JAr choriocarcinoma mother of blood type A and her offspring, also blood type A, in the cytotoxicity assay. The mother, who remains in complete remission, shows toxicity and recognition without blocking, as does the child of that pregnancy.

DISCUSSION

There is a chronologic evolution of immune reactivity during intrauterine and postnatal gestational life. Immunoglobulin (Ig) or B-cell development is believed to play an important role in the interaction and regulatory role of T- and B-cells. The major Ig in utero is IgG obtained from the mother through placental transfer. This globulin, detectable early in the first trimester, peaks about the 20th week and remains steady through delivery. The production of antibody within the fetus, as distinguished from the Ig that is transferred from the mother, is mainly in the form of IgM. IgM is detectable in the serum about the 20th week. If one utilizes in vitro culture fetal cells and measures capacity to produce Igs, fetal IgM appears as early as 10.5 weeks of gestation and IgG is noted at 12 weeks. The persistence of the initial reaction in the fetus of IgM as the permanent immunological response is in contrast with the adult, in whom IgM is only the primary response. Later, within a week or so it is superseded by predominant IgG response. However, IgM response in the fetus may persist through delivery and well into the postnatal period.

As it has been identified that malignancy in the placenta can exist during gestation, it is reasonable to conclude that initial fetal sensitization to choriocarcinoma tumor-associated antigens begins at that time. Maturation of immune competence in the fetus may be a determinant in the outcome of sensitization sufficient to protect the fetus from invasion by malignant choriocarcinoma cells. It might be speculated that the earlier the malignant transformation, the less the capacity of the placenta and fetus for mounting an effective immune response. Such an event might lead to unopposed invasion of malignant choriocarci noma cell transplacentally to the fetus. Difference in immunological response in the infant that died of metastatic choriocarcinoma and all other disease-free infants may relate to the point in time at which the malignant transformation occurred. Because transplantation antigens present in the fetus are generally localized on the plasma membrane and host cells are programed to reject foreign tissue, cells similar to transplant rejection phenomena may be expressed through the cytotoxic T-cells identified in this study. The mechanism of generation or time of generation during the intrauterine or postnatal periods are not known; however, the general principle of generation of diverse antigen-binding cells in bone marrow and thymus and their seeding in specific microenvironments in lymph nodes and spleen sets the stage for necessary antigen processing by macrophages. This processing may bring about sufficient antigen preparation suited for T- and B-cell interaction and ultimate generation of active progenitors with killer cell and immunocytotoxic properties. Careful dissection of the process of development of immune resistance of cells to neoplastic antigens will require complex models for which the trophoblast cell system may be well suited. Mechanisms for handling response to infectious agents including bacteria and viruses may likewise be investigated in such systems. At this point these initial data point to the exciting potential for new information in the field of placental and fetal immunology.

CONCLUSION

The offspring of postgestational choriocarcinoma mothers were examined for susceptibility or resistance to the malignancies of their placental cells. Three questions were asked: 1) Did their lymphocytes become sensitized to the malignancy during intrauterine gestation? 2) Did their lymphocytes retain the memory of this event? and 3) Have their lymphocytes retained cytotoxicity to the choriocarcinoma, thus affording resistance to choriocarcinoma? The results provided affirmative answers to each question. In all cases possible, the mother's choriocarcinoma was grown in tissue culture and lymphocytes from the mother and child were incubated to determine their recognition and cytotoxic capacity to kill these malignant cells from their own placenta, as well as from other patients with malignant trophoblastic disease. Two of the mothers died from resistant widespread disease; one of the children died of metastatic choriocarcinoma at 5 months of age; 15 of 18 high-risk mothers are in remission. All normal children and mothers in remission showed cytotoxicity to choriocarcinoma cells without blocking factor activity. The children were studied at 2, 3, 4, 5, and 10 years and were shown to have normal cytotoxicity at these critical points in their immunocompetence development.

REFERENCES

1. Ariel IM, Pack GT: Cancer and Allied Diseases of Infancy and Childhood. Little, Brown, Boston, 1960.
2. Brewer JI, Gerbie AB: Early development of choriocarcinoma. Am J Obstet Gynecol 94: 692, 1966.
3. Buckell EWC, Owen TK: Chorionepithelioma in mother and infant. J Obstet Gynaecol Br Emp 61: 329, 1954.
4. Daamen DBF, Bloem GWD, Westerbeck AJ: Chorionepithelioma in mother and child. J Obstet Gynaecol Br Comm 68: 144, 1961.
5. Driscoll SG: Choriocarcinoma: An "incidental finding" within a term placenta. Obstet Gynecol 21: 96, 1963.
6. Emery JL: Chorionepithelioma in a newborn male child with hyperplasia of the interstitial cells of the testes. J Pathol Bacteriol 64: 735, 1952.
7. Kay S, Reed WG: Chorioepithelioma of the lung in a female infant seven months old. Am J Pathol 29: 555, 1953.
8. Mercer RD, Lammert AC, Anderson R, Hazard JB: Choriocarcinoma in mother and infant. JAMA 166: 482, 1958.
9. Novak E, Seah C: Choriocarcinoma of uterus: Study of 74 cases from Mathieu memorial chorioepithelioma registry. Am J Obstet Gynecol 67: 933–961, 1954.
10. Pattillo RA, Gey G: Establishment of a cell line of human hormone-synthesizing trophoblastic cells in vitro. Cancer Res 28: 1231–1236, 1968.
11. Pattillo RA, Story MT, Ruckert ACF: Expression of cell-mediated immunity and blocking factor using a new line of ovarian cancer cells in vitro. Cancer Res 39: 1185–1191, 1979.

PART THREE

ENDOCRINOLOGY AND EPIDEMIOLOGY OF TROPHOBLASTIC DISEASES

8

Determination of Serum Trophoblastic Proteins in Diagnosis and Management of Trophoblastic Diseases

Noriaki Sakuragi

INTRODUCTION

After introduction of the concept of primary chemotherapy for patients with trophoblastic diseases, many cases have been treated with chemotherapy alone, even if a histological diagnosis has not been determined [3, 6]. However, this method has failed to obtain complete remission in some cases due to the considerable variation in the malignant potential of the invasive mole and choriocarcinoma. Thus, differentiation using a scoring system, of which the clinical availability has been evaluated, was designed independently by Ishizuka [4], Bagshawe [1], and Hammond et al. [2]. Data of whole-molecule human chorionic gonadotropin (hCG) has been included in these scoring systems.

Recent advances in endocrinology concerning trophoblastic proteins have enhanced the possibility that differentiation in the diagnosis of trophoblastic diseases would be performed by the measurement of trophoblastic proteins. In fact, the clinical availability of data from whole-molecule hCG, hCG-α subunit, hCG-β subunit, SP_1, and PP5 as the tumor marker has been described elsewhere in the literature. In this report, the significance of hCG-β and SP_1 values in differential diagnosis and in evaluation of responsiveness to chemotherapy will be discussed.

MATERIAL AND METHODS

Serum samples were obtained from 15 women with choriocarcinoma, 11 with invasive mole, 13 with complete hydatidiform mole, 6 with partial hydatidiform mole, and 21 normal women volunteers in various gestational weeks. Sampling was performed before initiation of treatment for trophoblastic diseases. Histological diagnosis as to whether the patients had choriocarcinoma or invasive mole was confirmed by the pathological findings of surgically resected specimens.

The serum SP_1 and hCG-β radioimmunoassay was performed with the use of a radioimmunoassay system produced by Behringwerke AG, West Germany and CIS, France, respectively, as described earlier [1]. Cross-reactivity with whole-molecule hCG in this hCG-β assay system was 6.7%. Assayed hCG-β levels are the sum total of free hCG-β and cross-reacted whole-molecule hCG. The intraassay and interassay coefficients of variation in SP_1 radioimmunoassay were 5.7% and 6.6%, respectively. The intraassay and interaassay coefficients of variation in hCG-β radioimmunoassay were 6.5% and 4.9%, respectively. Both protein levels are represented in nanograms per milliliter.

In addition to serum SP_1 and hCG-β levels, SP_1/hCG-β ratios that are nondimensional values were examined in order to eliminate the influence of the size of the trophoblastic mass.

RESULTS

Serum SP_1 and hCG-β Levels in Complete and Partial Hydatidiform Moles

Serum SP_1 level in complete mole was 15,743.1±15,273.0 (mean±SD) ng/mL; in partial mole it was 18,222.7±31,078.7 ng/mL. Serum hCG-β levels in complete mole and partial mole were 2417.1±1940.7 ng/mL and 353.8±538.9 ng/mL, respectively. SP_1/hCG-β ratios in complete mole and partial mole were 9.74±7.28 and 157.2±213.0, respectively. There is no significant difference in serum SP_1 levels, whereas hCG-β levels are significantly higher in the complete mole ($p<0.05$), and SP_1/hCG-β ratios are significantly higher in the partial mole ($p<0.05$) (Figure 1).

Changes in serum SP_1 and hCG-β levels after evacuation of moles were examined.

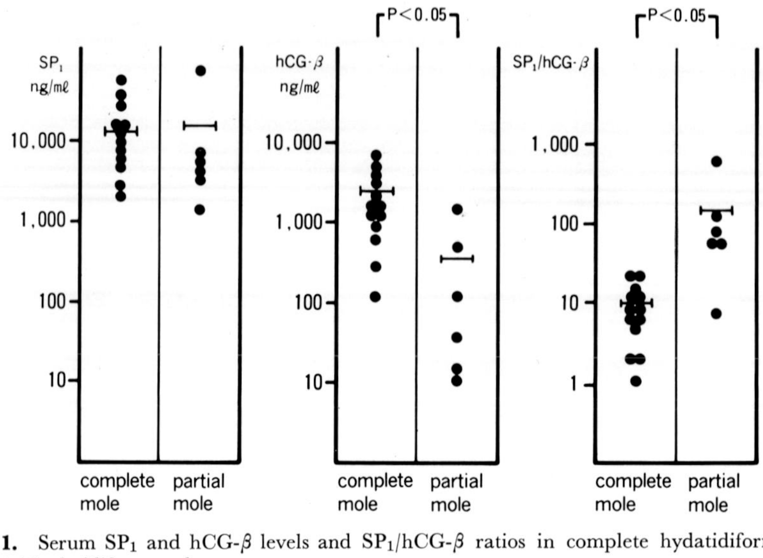

Figure 1. Serum SP_1 and hCG-β levels and SP_1/hCG-β ratios in complete hydatidiform mole and partial hydatidiform mole.

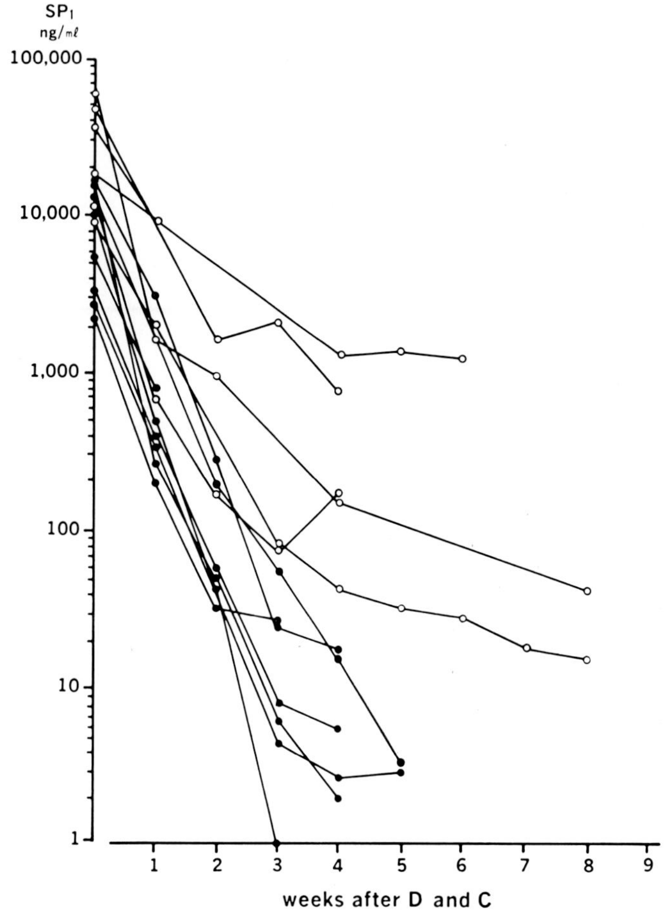

Figure 2. Changes in serum SP_1 levels after evacuation of hydatidiform mole: ○—○, with postmolar trophoblastic disease; ●—●, without postmolar trophoblastic disease.

Serum SP_1 levels at 4 weeks after evacuation were more than 40 ng/mL in those cases that had persistent trophoblastic diseases (Figure 2). Serum hCG-β levels at 4 weeks after evacuation were more than 20 ng/mL in those cases with persistent trophoblastic diseases (Figure 3).

Serum SP_1 and hCG-β Levels in Choriocarcinoma and Invasive Mole

Serum SP_1 levels in choriocarcinoma and invasive mole ranged from 2.9 to 3,050 (652.1 ± 911.6) ng/mL and from 8.2 to 3,051 (667.2 ± 953.1) ng/mL, respectively (Figure 4). Serum hCG-β levels ranged from 33.0 to 12,400 ($1{,}817.9 \pm 3{,}155.7$) ng/mL and from 8.2 to 1,780 (345.5 ± 531.7) ng/mL, respectively (Figure 5). There is no difference in serum SP_1 and hCG-β levels between choriocarcinoma and invasive mole.

SP_1/hCG-β ratios in choriocarcinoma and invasive mole were distributed between 0.06 and 0.96 (0.36 ± 0.26) and between 1.00 and 4.57 (2.10 ± 1.06), respectively. The ratios in choriocarcinoma are significantly lower than in invasive mole ($p < 0.001$). The ratios in choriocarcinoma are less than 1.0, whereas the ratios in invasive mole are 1.0 or more (Figure 6).

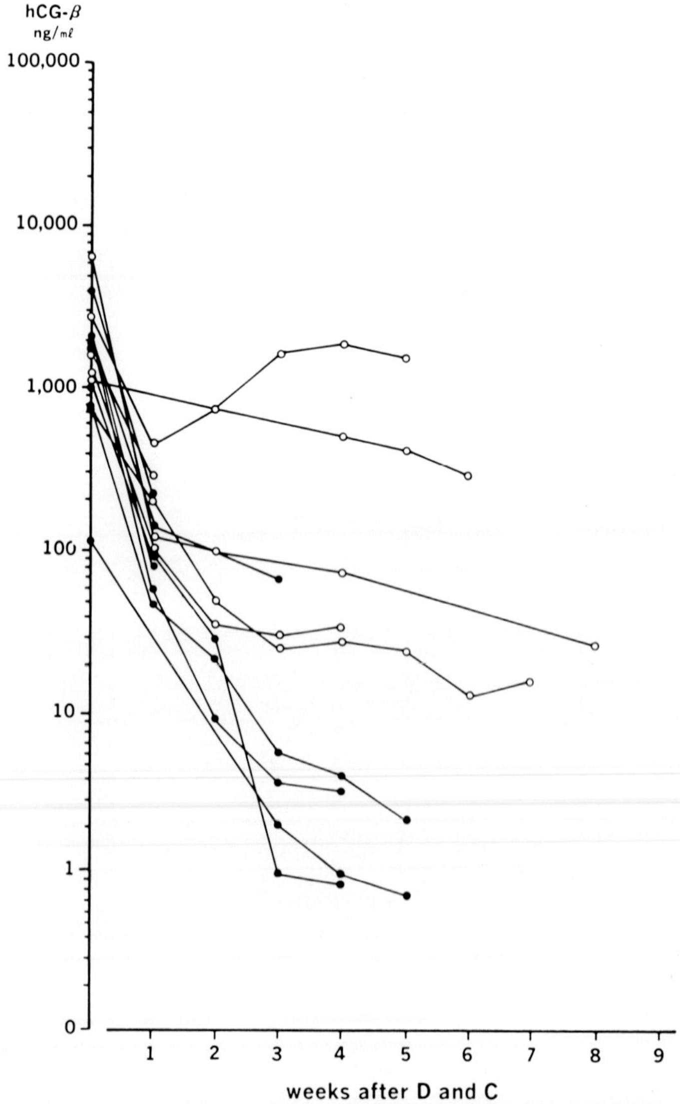

Figure 3. Changes in serum hCG-β levels after evacuation of hydatidiform mole: ○—○, with postmolar trophoblastic disease; ●—●, without postmolar trophoblastic disease.

SP$_1$ hCG-β Ratios in Choriocarcinoma, Invasive Mole, Complete Mole, and Normal Pregnancy in Various Gestational Weeks

The ratios in choriocarcinoma were lowest. In normal pregnancy, the ratio in the peri-implantation period is very low (under 0.48), which corresponds to that in choriocarcinoma. The ratio increases as the pregnancy progresses, and then reaches very high values (1,400–14,000) in the third trimester (Figure 7).

Changes in SP$_1$/hCG-β Ratios after Chemotherapy in Metastatic Choriocarcinoma Patients

Choriocarcinoma patients with metastases were divided into two groups: those who achieved complete remission, and those who died of the disease.

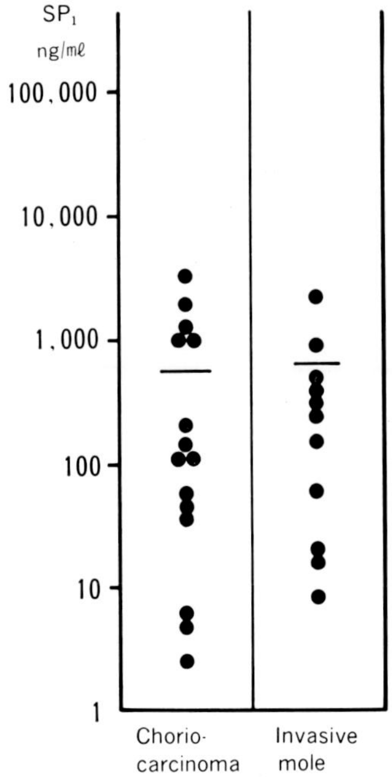

Figure 4. Serum SP_1 levels in choriocarcinoma and invasive mole. There is no statistically significant difference.

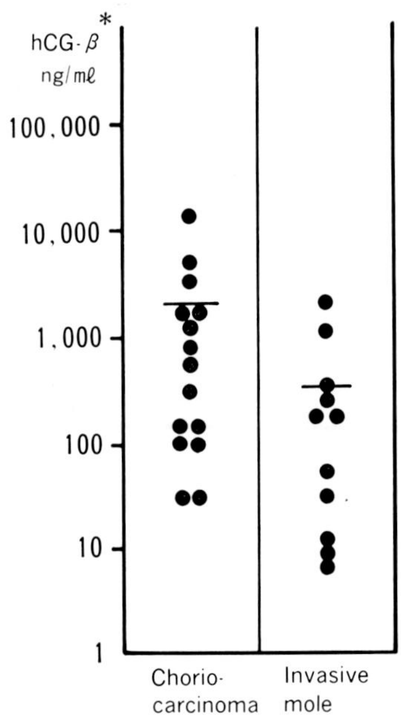

Figure 5. Serum hCG-β levels in choriocarcinoma and invasive mole. There is no statistically significant difference.

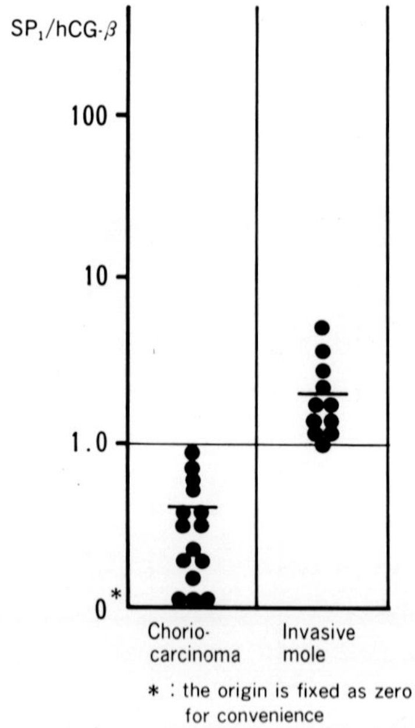

Figure 6. SP_1/hCG-β ratios in choriocarcinoma and invasive mole. There is a statistically significant difference ($p<0.001$).

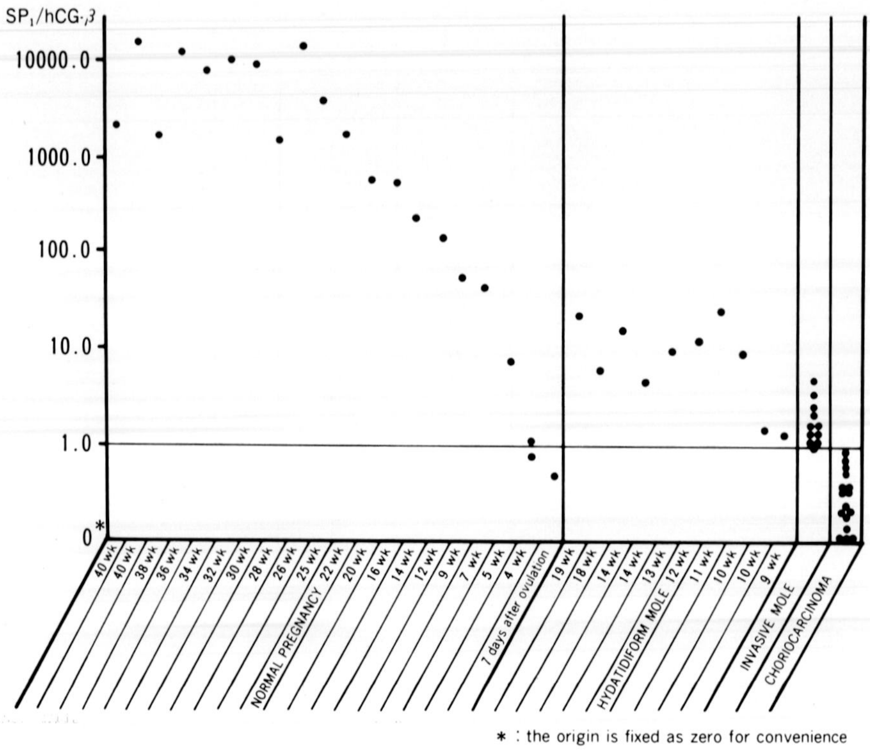

Figure 7. SP_1/hCG-β ratios in choriocarcinoma, invasive mole, hydatidiform mole, and normal pregnancy in various gestational weeks.

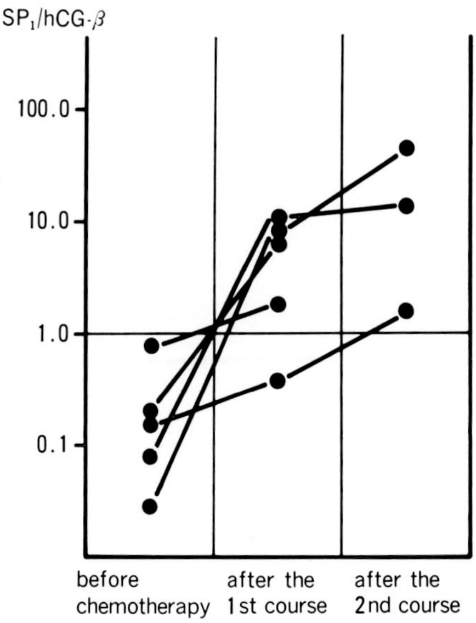

Figure 8. Changes in SP_1/hCG-β ratios after chemotherapy in metastatic choriocarcinoma patients who achieved complete remission.

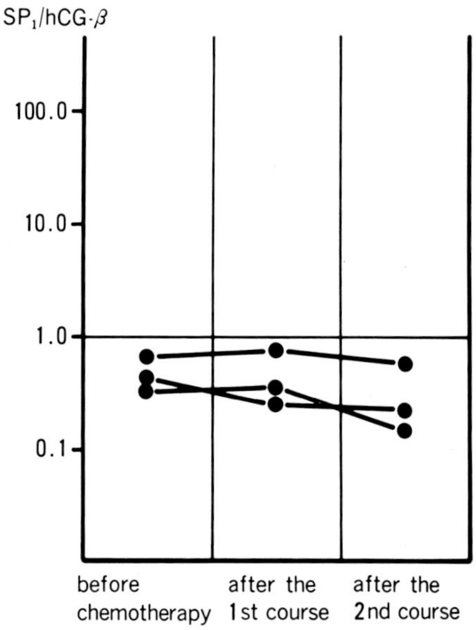

Figure 9. Changes in SP_1/hCG-β ratios after chemotherapy in metastatic choriocarcinoma patients who died of the disease.

The changes in the ratios after chemotherapy were compared between the two groups. In the remission group, the ratios increased after chemotherapy. In two of the five patients, marker protein levels decreased to a nondetectable level after the second course of chemotherapy (Figure 8). In those who died of the disease, the ratio remained at low levels (Figure 9). The ratios in metastatic invasive mole increased after chemotherapy. Chemotherapy was effective and all achieved remission (Figure 10).

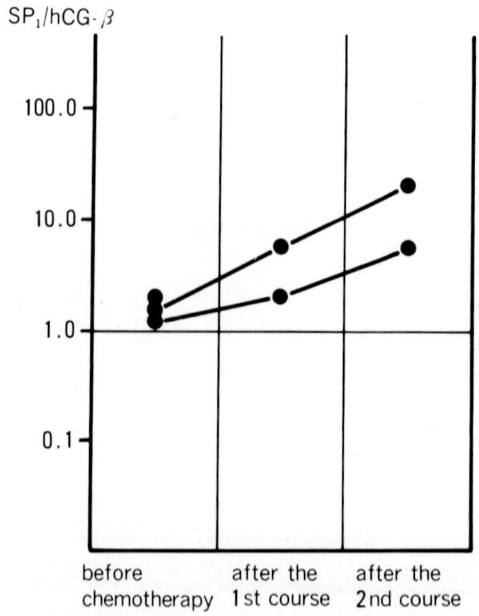

Figure 10. Changes in SP_1/hCG-β ratios after chemotherapy in metastatic invasive mole patients.

Table 1. Clinical data of two cases of metastatic choriocarcinoma

Patient	Age	Antecedent pregnancy	HCG at onset (mIU/mL)	Metastatic sites	Treatment regimen	Outcome
OJ	26	Term	32,000	Lung, liver	MTX, act-D	Complete remission
KM	30	Term	320,000	Lung, liver, vagina	MTX, act-D	Death of disease

MTX=methotrexate; act-D=actinomycin-D.

Two cases with choriocarcinoma and the changes in serum hCG-β levels and SP_1/hCG-β ratios are presented (Table 1). Both cases had term delivery as an antecedent pregnancy and had lung and liver metastases. Patient OJ achieved complete remission, whereas patient KM died of the disease. In both cases, serum hCG-β levels decreased after chemotherapy. However, the changes in SP_1/hCG-β ratios were different. The ratio increased after chemotherapy in OJ, but remained at a low level in KM (Figure 11).

DISCUSSION

Urinary or serum hCG or hCG-β levels have been determined to be tumor markers for trophoblastic disease monitoring. The possible clinical usefulness of other trophoblastic proteins in management of trophoblastic diseases has been discussed in many papers. It has been shown that the differential diagnosis between choriocarcinoma and invasive mole can be achieved by analyzing serum trophoblastic proteins [5, 7, 8].

From the data on serum SP_1 and hCG-β levels after evacuation of moles, SP_1 determination seems useful for detecting malignant sequelae after evacuation of moles. Invasive moles and postmolar choriocarcinomas usually originate from a complete mole. Malignant sequelae after partial mole is rare. Partial mole is distinguished from complete

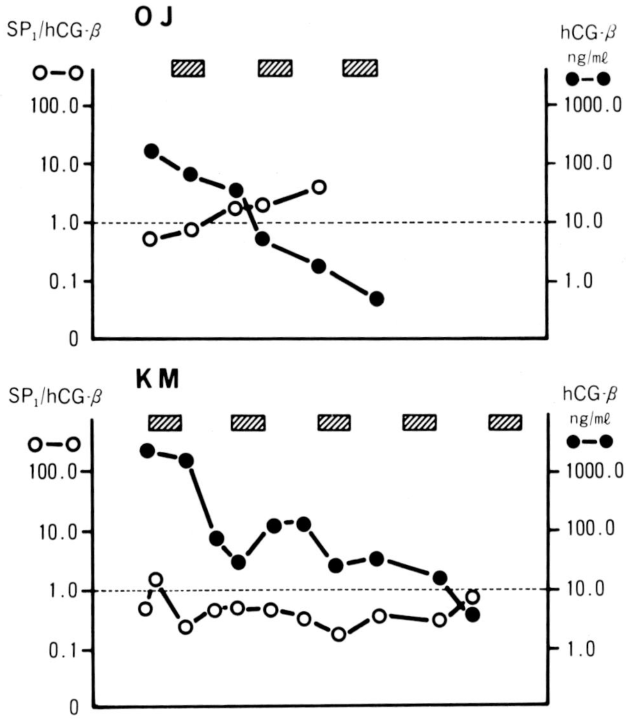

Figure 11. Changes in serum hCG-β levels and SP_1/hCG-β ratios in two cases of metastatic choriocarcinoma.

mole by its macroscopic appearance. Chromosomal differences between the two have been elucidated by many investigators. Serum SP_1 and hCG-β determination is useful to discriminate complete and partial moles, as shown in the results. SP_1/hCG-β ratio may be an important index to differentiate these two types of moles.

The data from this work suggest that the SP_1/hCG-β ratio may represent the degree of differentiation of trophoblasts. In postmolar trophoblastic diseases, SP_1/hCG-β ratio of 1.0 or more before treatment is indicative for invasive mole. A ratio under 1.0 is indicative for choriocarcinoma. However, serum SP_1 and hCG-β levels at the time when the levels are steadily falling after evacuation of mole should not be used for determination of the ratio.

It is well known that chemotherapeutic agents effective for choriocarcinoma can induce differentiation of trophoblastic cells. So it may be expected that, after chemotherapy, the ratio in choriocarcinoma sensitive to the drugs will exhibit characteristic changes different from those in choriocarcinoma refractory to chemotherapy. The results suggest that the changes in SP_1/hCG-β ratio in choriocarcinoma patients after chemotherapy seem to represent the effectiveness of the therapy or patients' prognosis. When the ratio increases over 1.0 after one or two courses of chemotherapy, a good prognosis can be expected. If it remains under 1.0 after one or two courses, a poor prognosis will follow.

SUMMARY

Serum SP_1 and hCG-β subunit (hCG-β) levels and SP_1/hCG-β ratios were determined for trophoblastic diseases and normal pregnancies. There was no significant difference in serum SP_1 and hCG-β levels between choriocarcinoma and invasive mole. The SP_1/hCG-β ratio in normal pregnancy was lowest at the period of implantation (under 0.48). The ratio increased with the gestational week. It reached its greatest value (1,400–14,000) in the third trimester. The ratio in choriocarcinoma was low (0.36 ± 0.26), which was consistent with normal pregnant women in the periimplantation period. The ratio in invasive mole was 2.10 ± 1.06, which is significantly higher than in choriocarcinoma.

Changes in the SP_1/hCG-β ratio after chemotherapy in eight cases with metastatic choriocarcinoma were examined. The ratio increased to over 1.0 after one or two courses of chemotherapy in five or eight patients. These cases achieved complete remission. The ratio remained below 1.0 in the other three patients, who died of the disease.

These results suggest that serum SP_1/hCG-β ratio is one of the important indices predicting the prognosis of choriocarcinoma patients.

REFERENCES

1. Bagshawe KD: Risk and prognostic factors in trophoblastic neoplasia. Cancer 38: 1373, 1976.
2. Hammond CB, Borchert LG, Tyey L, Creasman WT, Parker RT: Treatment of metastatic trophoblastic disease: Good and poor prognosis. Am J Obstet Gynecol 115: 451, 1973.
3. Hertz R, Lewis J, Lipsett MB: Five years' experience with the chemotherapy of metastatic choriocarcinoma and related trophoblastic tumors in women. Am J Obstet Gynecol 82: 631, 1961.
4. Ishizuka N: Diagnosis and therapy of destructive hydatidiform mole and chorionepithelioma. Nippon Sanka Fujinka Gakkai Zasshi 21: 1443, 1969.
5. Lee JN, Salem HT, Al-Ani AT, Chard T, Huang SC, Ouyang PC, Wei PY, Seppälä M: Circulating concentration of specific placental proteins (human chorionic gonadotropin, pregnancy-specific beta-1 glycoprotein, and placental protein 5) in untreated gestational trophoblastic tumors. Am J Obstet Gynecol 139: 702, 1981.
6. Li MD, Hertz R, Spencer DB: Effects of methotrexate upon choriocarcinoma and chorioadenoma. Proc Soc Exp Biol Med 93: 361, 1956.
7. Sakuragi N: Serum SP_1 and hCG-β subunit (hCG-β) levels in choriocarcinoma, invasive mole and hydatidiform mole—clinical significance of SP_1/hCG-β ratio. Gynecol Oncol 13: 393, 1982.
8. Yazaki K, Yazaki C, Wakabayashi K, Igarashi M: Iso-electric heterogeneity of human chorionic gonadotropin: Presence of choriocarcinoma specific components. Am J Obstet Gynecol 138: 189, 1980.

9

Endocrinological Status and Malignant Progression Following Hydatidiform Mole in Elderly Patients over 40 Years of Age

Hiroaki Soma, Kenichi Okudera, Masaomi Takayama,
and Shizuko Yamabe

INTRODUCTION

It is generally agreed that the incidence of hydatidiform mole is extremely high in elderly women over 40 years of age, whereas the absolute number of pregnancies achieved by older women greatly diminishes [8]. The risk of subsequent malignant progression after removal of the mole is significantly higher in elderly patients than in younger patients [2, 5, 6, 8]. The present paper discusses a relationship between endocrinological status and malignant progression after removal of hydatidiform mole in elderly women over 40 years of age.

MATERIALS AND METHODS

From 1974 to 1984, the records of 39 patients over 40 years of age with hydatidiform moles at Tokyo Medical College Hospital were analyzed. All records were reviewed noting details of premolar diagnosis, malignant sequelae, human chorionic gonadotropin [hCG] titer at diagnosis, the slope of hCG regression after removal of the mole, chemotherapy, and outcome. After evacuation of the mole, serial determinations of hCG (by hCG titration technique, Kyorin, and Higonavis, Mochida), β-hCG (by radioimmunoassay [RIA]) and SP_1 (by RIA) were performed and compared in 28 patients over 40 years old and in 43 patients under 40 years old.

RESULTS

The age distribution of the 39 patients that were 40 to 54 years old consisted of 11 cases, over 50 years; 17 cases, 45 to 49 years; 11 cases, 40 to 44 years. Table 1 shows premolar diagnosis in elderly patients with hydatidiform mole. In elderly patients, pregnancy is often unexpected, so an accurate preoperative diagnosis is often mistaken. A diagnostic curettage is strongly indicated in cases of premenopausal or postmenopausal bleeding and is useful in the diagnosis of unsuspected trophoblastic disease. In this report, uterine evacuation of the mole was performed in 22 cases. Of the false diagnoses made, myoma uteri was the most common misdiagnosis, occurring in 14 cases. Three of nine cases diagnosed as hydatidiform mole following hysterectomy had an invasive mole in the myometrium. Although hysterectomy was the common surgical procedure in elderly women with hydatidiform mole, an ultrasound examination should be used before operation to avoid the possibility of menopause based on amenorrhea.

Table 2 shows the number of elderly patients who developed subsequent malignant progression following hydatidiform mole. Of 39 patients, 17 cases developed malignancies, including eight choriocarcinomas and nine invasive moles. Eight patients had pulmonary metastasis; thereafter two patients died of extensive metastases. Vaginal metastasis was noted in one patient. Other diseases such as nephrosis, severe toxemia, hepatitis, and dyspnea due to lung edema were complicated by hydatidiform mole.

Table 3 shows urinary hCG titers at the time of initial diagnosis of hydatidiform mole in 30 elderly patients. The titers ranged widely from 4,910,000 IU/liter to 2,400 IU/liter. Such wide ranges of hCG levels in elderly patients may be due to delayed measurements of hCG titers after evacuation of the mole.

Postmolar chemotherapy with MAC (methotrexate [MTX], actinomycin-D [act-D], cyclophosphamide) or MA plus NK-171 (VP-16, Etoposide) performed for 25 elderly

Table 1. Premolar diagnosis in elderly patients with hydatidiform mole

Procedure	No. of cases
D & C or evacuation	22
Hysterectomy	9 (Invasive mole 3)
Myoma uteri	14

D & C = dilatation and curettage.

Table 2. Malignant progression in elderly patients with hydatidiform mole

Outcome	No. of cases
Choriocarcinoma	8
Invasive mole	9
Undetermined	2
Lung metastasis	8
Vaginal metastasis	1
Death due to extensive metastases	2
Complicated by other disease	**No. of cases**
Nephrosis	1
Severe toxemia	1
Marked edema	
Hypertension	
Albuminuria	
Hepatitis	2
Dyspnea	3

Table 3. hCG titers at time of diagnosis of hydatidiform mole

hCG titer	No. of cases
≦2,400 IU/liter	7
≦9,600 IU/liter	4
≦32,000 IU/liter	2
≦76,800 IU/liter	2
≦153,600 IU/liter	4
≦256,000 IU/liter	3
≦409,600 IU/liter	3
≦819,200 IU/liter	3
≦4,910,000 IU/liter	2

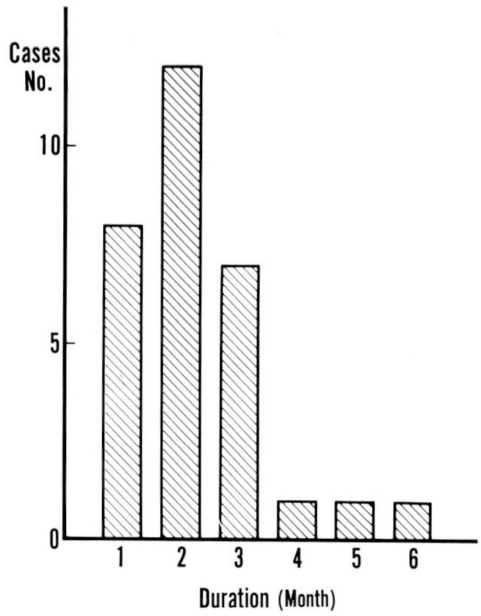

Figure 1. Duration until hCG titer fell to LH levels following chemotherapy.

patients ranged from two to seven courses, except for one case with distant metastasis that received ten courses. The hCG levels in elderly patients on admission to the hospital ranged widely. It took about 2 to 6 months until the hCG titers fell to luteinizing hormone (LH) level even while chemotherapy was being given (Figure 1). When the hCG titer did not fall to the LH level because of higher pituitary gonadotropin secretion in perimenopausal state or suspected malignant progression, simultaneous measurements of another placental protein, SP_1, is helpful for determination.

In the patient aged 52 years who had vulval metastasis after removal of a hydatidiform mole by hysterectomy, the urinary hCG level was 76,800 IU/liter, the serum SP_1 level was 15,458 ng/mL, and the serum β-hCG level was 546.2 ng/mL. Both hCG and SP_1 levels decreased during treatment with MTX and it took 72 days until SP_1 disappeared and the patient was in full clinical remission [9].

Figure 2 shows serial hCG values following surgical management in 12 elderly patients with trophoblastic disease. Although there were big differences in urinary hCG titers when the patients were admitted to the hospital, serial hCG levels gradually decreased during treatment. It took from about 35 to 55 days after treatment for the hCG value to decline below 100 IU/liter in six cases; two cases maintained low concentrations of hCG since hospitalization. It took from 65 to 95 days for the hCG level to decline to 100 IU/liter in four cases, whereas in a young patient with vaginal metastasis after hydati-

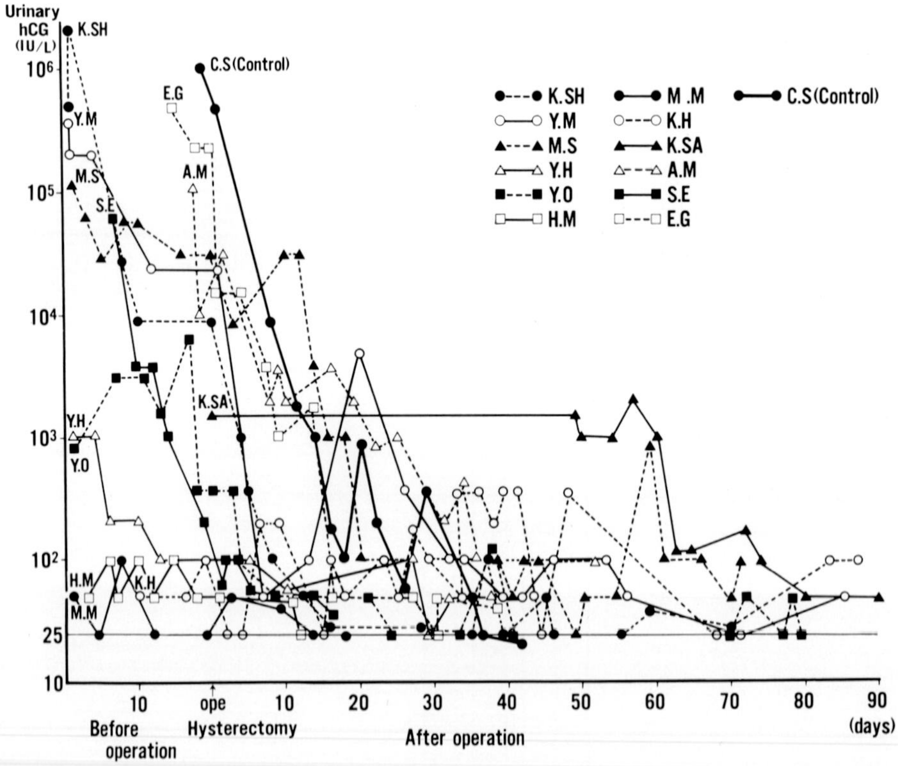

Figure 2. Serial hCG values following surgical management in elderly patients with trophoblastic disease.

diform mole, hCG titer fell below 25 IU/liter at about 40 days after removal of the mole. However, in six elderly patients including two with invasive moles, two with choriocarcinomas, and two with hydatidiform moles, hCG levels remained above 100 IU/liter even over 60 days after treatment.

Mean hCG concentrations for 28 patients with trophoblastic disease over 40 years of age and 43 patients under 40 years of age were compared. The weekly mean urinary hCG values after evacuation of the hydatidiform mole in both groups declined below 100 IU/liter from 4 to 8 weeks, whereas the mean titer of hCG tended only to decline to 1,000 IU/liter at about 8 weeks after treatment in both groups who developed subsequent malignant progression. The mean concentration of serum hCG-β after treatment in both patients with trophoblastic disease showed similar declining tendencies with pattern of urinary hCG levels (Figure 3). The mean serum SP_1 concentrations in both groups exhibited considerable clear-cut decline from 4 to 8 weeks in the group over 40 years of age with hydatidiform mole and invasive mole (Figure 4).

These figures show a decline in hCG, hCG-β, and SP_1 concentrations following evacuation of mole, suggesting that simultaneous measurements of placental proteins in trophoblastic disease can be used to determine the risk of malignant sequelae following mole in women over 40 years of age and younger. This is true despite the unexpected data showing that there were no significant changes in hCG titers between both groups.

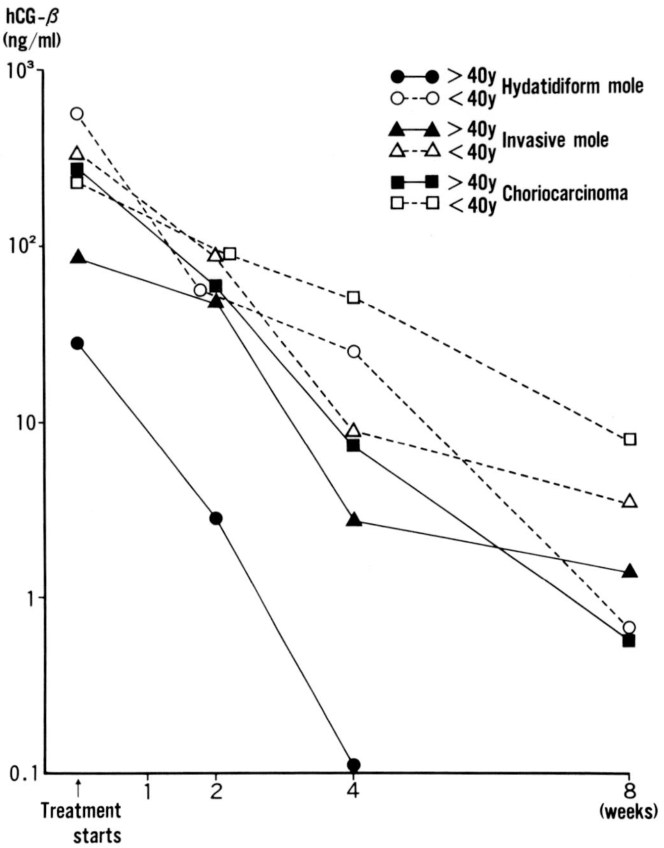

Figure 3. A comparison of mean hCG-β levels between patients with trophoblastic disease over 40 years old and those under 40 years old.

Case 1

A 54-year-old woman, gravida 5, para 2, was admitted to Funabashi City Medical Center with complaints of generalized edema, dyspnea, hypertension, proteinuria, abdominal tumor mass, and slight genital bleeding. The patient underwent hysterectomy 21 days after admission. The uterus revealed complete hydatidiform mole with invasive mole, and bilateral pulmonary metastases were found on chest film. The patient was transferred to our hospital 1 month later. On admission, hCG titer was 2,500 IU/liter. However, hCG levels remained over 1,000 IU/liter for over 60 days. After five courses of chemotherapy with MTX, act-D, and NK-171, hCG fell to LH levels and pulmonary metastases disappeared.

The uterine specimen that had been removed showed the area of the myometrium invaded by mole (Figure 5). Histologically deported villi in the vessel of the myometrium were also identified.

Case 2

A 42-year-old patient, para 2, with complete mole of estimated 10 weeks gestation showed 3,276,800 IU/liter of hCG. The hCG titer decreased below 40 IU/liter for 3 months after evacuation of the mole. However, 4 months later, her hCG elevated again to 320 IU/liter. After chemotherapy with NK-171, her hCG level fell to 25 IU/liter for 2

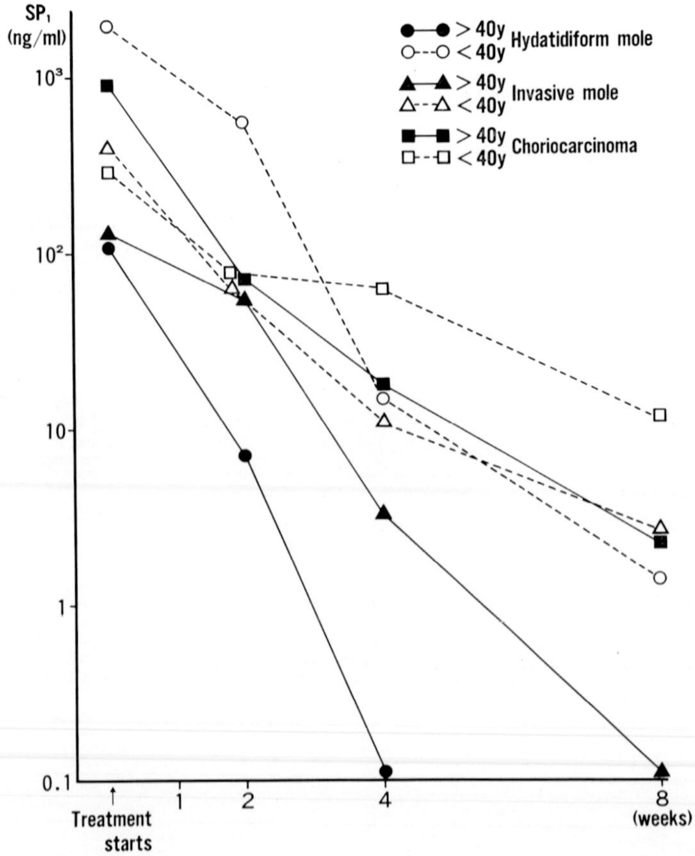

Figure 4. A comparison of mean SP_1 levels between patients with trophoblastic disease over 40 years old and those under 40 years old.

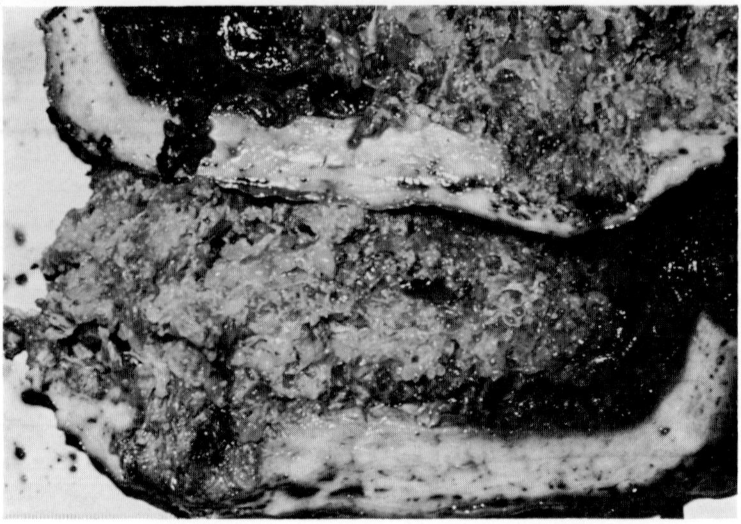

Figure 5. Case 1. The area of the myometrium invaded by mole.

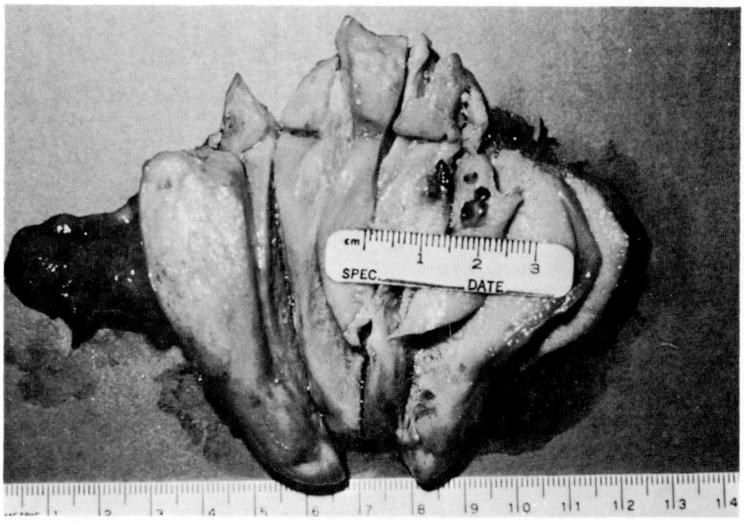

Figure 6. Case 2. Small tumor foci were found in the left corner of the myometrium.

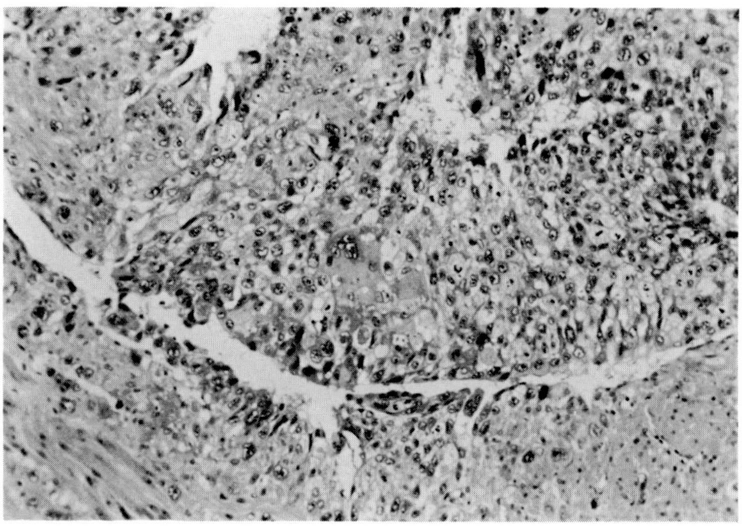

Figure 7. Case 3. Histologic diagnosis was choriocarcinoma. (Original magnification × 100.)

months. A hysterectomy was then performed. A focus of 0.5 × 0.3 cm in size was found in the left corner of the myometrium (Figure 6). The histologic findings showed mass of trophoblastic cells in the myometrium. Thereafter, hCG level remained below 25 IU/liter.

Case 3

A 49-year-old patient, para 3, who has received treatment for hepatitis since 1969, complained of massive genital bleeding. She presented with her uterus as large as a fetal head. A sonogram revealed molar gestation, and hCG titer showed 5,122,000 IU/liter. After evacuation of the complete mole, pelvic angiography revealed abnormal staining in the right corner of the uterus. Serum hCG level was 15,000 mIU/mL, and serum SP_1 level

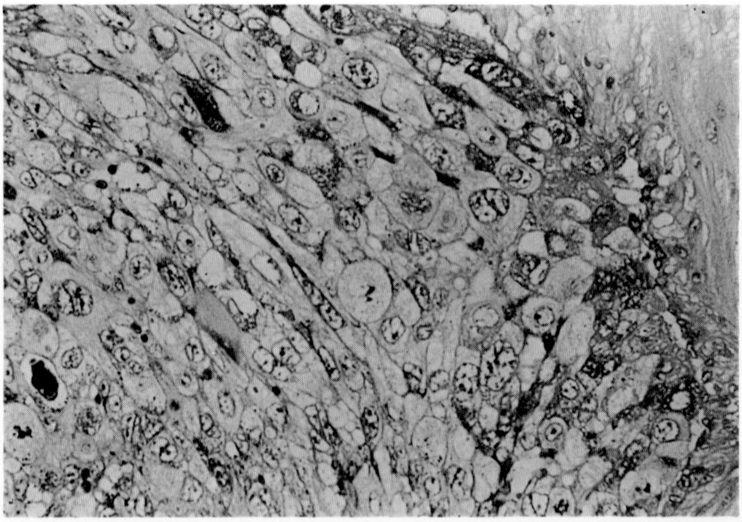

Figure 8. Case 3. Choriocarcinoma cell mass embolized in the vessel of the myometrium. (PAS stain, original magnification ×200.)

Table 4. Prognosis of postmolar treatment for elderly patients

Good prognosis—duration	No.	Relapse—duration	No.
6 mo	7	3 mo	1
1 yr	5	2 yr	1
2 yr	4	5 yr	1
3 yr	3		
4 yr	4		
5 yr	3		
6 yr	1		
10 yr	1		

was 520 ng/mL. Chemotherapy with MAC was given and hysterectomy was performed. In the right corner of the uterine fundus, tumor foci were found. The histologic diagnosis was choriocarcinoma (Figure 7), and choriocarcinoma cell mass was embolized in the vessel of the myometrium (Figure 8). A chromosome study showed 46,XX with quinacrine and Giemsa-banding techniques. Thereafter hCG level fell to 50 IU/liter. No metastasis was found in the lung.

Even after chemotherapy has been given for a long duration following removal of mole, small tumor foci often remain in the uterus of some patients who have undergone hysterectomy. Table 4 shows the outcome of postmolar treatment for 31 elderly patients with trophoblastic disease. There was a good prognosis in 28 cases, but three cases developed relapse or metastases of choriocarcinoma from 3 months to 5 years after treatment, and two died of extensive metastases.

DISCUSSION

Starting at the age of 40 years, the incidence of ovulatory cycles rapidly diminishes; therefore, the chance of pregnancy gradually diminishes. However, the risk of developing trophoblastic disease following pregnancy is greatly increased beyond the age of 40 years when compared with the risk for pregnancies under the age of 39 years [1, 5]. Accordingly, age-specific rates of hydatidiform mole have identified as a J-shaped curve [4, 8]. At the same time, in elderly patients over 40 years of age, the rate of malignant sequelae after hydatidiform mole is extremely high when compared with that in younger patients.

According to our previous information [8], the incidence of hydatidiform mole showed a 45-fold increase in 27 patients over 45 years of age. About 66% of them developed subsequently a malignant progression such as invasive mole and choriocarcinoma. The present results thus confirm previous reports showing a high incidence of malignant sequelae following hydatidiform mole.

In elderly patients, pregnancy is often unexpected. The diagnosis may therefore be mistaken. Most of the patients had a history of irregular menses or amenorrhea before hydatidiform mole, so there was a tendency for misdiagnoses as menopause or dysfunctional bleeding. Of the false diagnoses made, leiomyoma uteri was the most common misdiagnosis. When initial hysterectomy for myoma uteri exposed often complete hydatidiform mole, invasive moles were found in 33% of the myometrium. Accordingly, an ultrasound examination and hCG determinations should be used before operation to avoid the possibility of misdiagnosis.

According to Lurain et al. [7], approximately 20% of patients with hydatidiform mole will require treatment after evacuation. However, elderly patients with hydatidiform mole require extra attention regarding serial hCG determination, subsequent malignant progression, and postmolar chemotherapy. Urinary hCG levels in elderly patients with hydatidiform mole on admission to hospital ranged widely, and it took about 2 to 6 months until hCG titers fell to LH levels even while chemotherapy was being given. A greater increase of pituitary gonadotropin in elderly patients who have undergone hysterectomy with bilateral oophorectomy at perimenopausal state is strongly suggested. When hCG titer does not fall to LH level, hypergonadotropin titer or suspected malignant progression should be therefore considered in elderly women over the age of 40 years.

Pregnancy-specific β-glycoprotein (SP_1) was first isolated and purified from the human placenta and is synthesized by the trophoblast [3]. According to our previous report [9], after removal of hydatidiform moles, urinary hCG, β-hCG, and SP_1 levels were similar, but SP_1 levels tended to exceed serum β-hCG levels and SP_1 usually disappeared first. The SP_1 level is not influenced by hypersecretion of pituitary gonadotropin. Accordingly, coincident simultaneous measurements of SP_1 with hCG and β-hCG will be useful in the monitoring of elderly patients being treated for trophoblastic disease.

Even after chemotherapy was given for long duration following removal of mole and hCG remained at a low level, small tumor foci often remained in the uterus of some patients who underwent hysterectomy. In an elderly patient with hydatidiform mole, choriocarcinoma was found in the uterus, which was removed only 17 days after evacuation of the mole.

Although the present study showed a significant good prognosis in the outcome of postmolar treatment for 31 elderly patients with trophoblastic disease, three cases developed relapse or metastases of choriocarcinoma after 3 months to 5 years. Thus, these elderly patients over 40 years of age have a greater risk of postmolar trophoblastic disease and need to be considered for careful treatment of long duration.

CONCLUSION

The incidence of hydatidiform mole in elderly women over 40 years of age is extremely high. At the same time, in elderly patients who have hydatidiform mole, the risk of choriocarcinoma or invasive mole after removal of hydatidiform mole is significantly higher than in the younger group.

This report discussed endocrinological status and malignant progression. The age distribution of the 39 patients that were 40 to 54 years old consisted of 11 cases over 50 years; 17 cases, 45 to 49 years; and 11 cases, 40 to 44 years. Of 39 patients, 17 cases developed eight choriocarcinomas and nine invasive moles. Eight patients had pulmonary metastasis; thereafter two patients died of extensive metastases. Although hCG levels in 30 elderly patients on admission to hospital ranged widely, it took about 2 to 6 months until hCG titers fell to LH level, even while chemotherapy was being given. When hCG titer did not fall to LH level because of higher pituitary gonadotropin secretion in perimenopausal state or suspected malignant progression, simultaneous measurement of another placental protein, SP_1, is helpful for determination. Furthermore, even after chemotherapy was given for long duration following removal of the mole, small tumor foci often remained in the uterus of some patients who underwent hysterectomy.

In conclusion, hydatidiform mole in elderly patients over 40 years of age has an increased risk of choriocarcinoma or invasive mole. Therefore, careful management of these patients is indicated.

REFERENCES

1. Bagshawe KD: Risk and prognostic factors in trophoblastic neoplasia. Cancer 38: 1373–1385, 1976.
2. Bandy LC, Clarke-Pearson DL, Hammond CB: Malignant potential of gestational trophoblastic disease at the extreme ages of reproductive life. Obstet Gynecol 64: 395–399, 1984.
3. Bohn H: Nachweis und Charakterisierung von Schwangerschaftsproteinen in der menschlichen Plazenta, so wie ihre quantitative immunologische Bestimmung im Serum Schwanger Frauen. Arch Gynäkol 210: 440–457, 1971.
4. Grimes DA: Epidemiology of gestational trophoblastic disease. Am J Obstet Gynecol 150: 309–318, 1984.
5. Ichinoe K, Okada Y, Mabuchi Y, Yokota H, Kanamaru H: Incidence of hydatidiform mole and subsequent chorionic disease in reference to maternal age (in Japanese). Acta Obstet Gynaecol Jpn 31: 192–198, 1979.
6. Jequir AM, Winterton WR: Diagnostic problems of trophoblastic disease in women aged 50 or more. Obstet Gynecol 42: 378–387, 1973.
7. Lurain JR, Brewer JI, Torok EE, Holpern B: Natural history of hydatidiform mole after primary evacuation. Am J Obstet Gynecol 145: 591–595, 1983.
8. Soma H, Takayama M, Saito T, Isaka K: Management of hydatidiform mole in women over 45 years old. Asia-Oceania J Obstet Gynecol 9: 393–398, 1983.
9. Soma H, Kikuchi K, Takayama M, Saegusa H, Saito T, Kashiwagi H, Sayama S: Concentrations of SP_1 and β-HCG in serum and cerebrospinal fluid and concentrations of HCG in urine in patients with trophoblastic tumour. Arch Gynecol 230: 321–327, 1981.

10

Choriocarcinoma and Placental Protein Hormones

Matsuto Mochizuki, Takeshi Maruo, Makoto Hoshina, and Ryuichiro Nishimura

INTRODUCTION

Human trophoblast produces two major protein hormones, human chorionic gonadotropin (hCG) and human placental lactogen (hPL). It is well known that in patients with trophoblastic disease a disproportionately low concentration of serum hPL is usually observed along with higher hCG levels [2, 15]. In particular, the serum hPL level in patients with choriocarcinoma is extremely low or undetectable. This marked dissociation of two protein hormones in the serum is characteristic of choriocarcinoma. Therefore, it appears that there is an aberrant expression of these hormonal genes in trophoblastic neoplasms. Furthermore, an alteration in the regulation of hCG synthesis in choriocarcinoma and structural changes in the sugar chains of choriocarcinoma hCG have been recently demonstrated.

Here we report our recent findings regarding 1) gene expression of hCG (α, β) and hPL in trophoblastic neoplasms, especially choriocarcinoma; 2) alteration in steroid modulation of hCG synthesis and secretion in choriocarcinoma; 3) alteration in structure of sugar chains of hCG in choriocarcinoma; and 4) clinical application of detection of malignant change of hCG sugar chains for the biochemical diagnosis of choriocarcinoma.

GENE EXPRESSION OF PLACENTAL PROTEIN HORMONES

Many immunohistochemical studies using specific antibodies have suggested that hPL and hCG-α and -β subunits are synthesized in the syncytiotrophoblasts, whereas other studies have indicated that cytotrophoblasts may contain the hCG-α subunit [3]. One would expect that the mRNA encoding the hormone would be present in the particular trophoblast where synthesis occurs.

Accordingly, to identify the cellular localization of these mRNAs and to assess the cytological changes of the mRNAs during placental development and differentiation, we performed in situ hybridization. The attractive feature of this method is that it allows detection of specific mRNAs in individual cells.

Sections of frozen placental tissue were hybridized to ^{3}H-labeled cDNA probes complementary to hCG-α, hCG-β, and hPLmRNA, and were then washed to remove unhybridized probes. The slides were coated with an emulsion and the signals of cDNA-mRNA hybrids were visualized by autoradiography.

With an hPL probe, the silver grains are confined only to the syncytial region. In addition, no significant grains are present over cytotrophoblasts. With hCG-α probe, the silver grains for hCG-αmRNA are localized to the syncytium. And in contrast to hPL, several grains are present over cytotrophoblasts [4].

To see the change of mRNA levels of each protein during pregnancy we measured mean grain count per nucleus in the autoradiogram with in situ hybridization. The levels of hCG-α and hCG-βmRNA per unit of syncytial mass decreased toward term, whereas the level of hPL was constant throughout pregnancy [7].

Therefore, the expression of the hPL gene is constitutive, and hPL protein level in the serum is in proportion to placental weight. The data presented here also imply that the expression of these peptides is well correlated to trophoblast differentiation.

In the case of choriocarcinoma, there were abundant messages for hCG-α and hCG-β on syncytiotrophoblastic cells. In contrast, with an hPL probe few signals were observed [5]. As choriocarcinoma showing vigorous proliferation consists of undifferentiated trophoblasts, we assume that the differentiation of the trophoblast has been blocked before the expression of hPL gene. These observations can be summarized as follows. The progeny of mitotically active mononucleated cytotrophoblast differentiate to mitotically inactive syncytiotrophoblast, probably through the intermediate cell. During this differentiation process, hCG expression occurs first, probably just before syncytial formation then hCG-β expression begins. In the well-differentiated syncytiotrophoblasts hPL expression occurs, and by this time α and β expression decrease significantly [8].

The other possible explanation for the low level of hPLmRNA in choriocarcinoma is gene deletion. To assess this, we extracted DNA from choriocarcinoma and analyzed with Southern blotting hybridizing to hPLcDNA. Because of a small amount of DNA in choriocarcinoma, the intensity of the bands was faint compared to DNAs of normal and hydatidiform mole tissue, but we still could observe an essentially identical pattern in each case. Therefore, the DNA sequences especially for the structural region of hPL in trophoblastic disease are essentially identical to those of normal DNA. Probably a low level of expression of hPL gene in choriocarcinoma is due to the disturbance of regulatory gene.

The mechanisms of the gene regulation for placental protein hormones are still unknown. One possible mechanism is methylation of cytosine, which is only one of modifications of nucleotide. Then we examined the level of cytosine methylation with methylation sensitive and nonsensitive restriction endonuclease, Hpa II and Msp I. There were clear differences in the restriction patterns of the DNA extracted from first trimester or term placenta. From these results, it was known that the methylation levels of cytosine in the vicinity of hCG-α, hCG-β, and hPL gene progress toward term. In other words, the

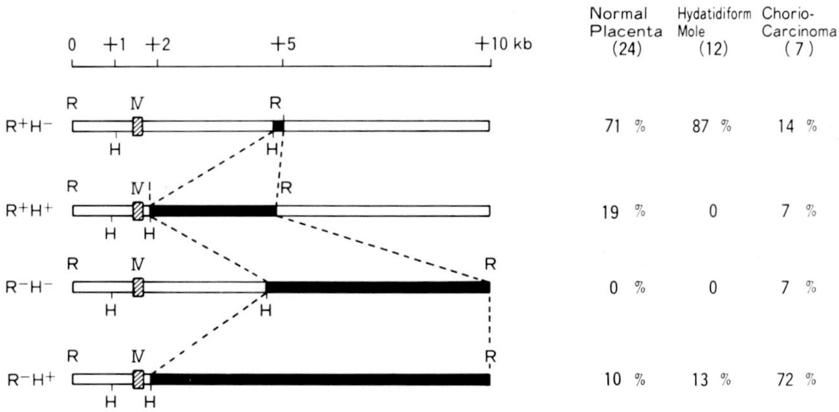

Figure 1. hCG-α gene polymorphisms in trophoblastic disease.

expression of hCG-α and hCG-β was suppressed by cytosine methylation, whereas hPL expression was unchanged.

Another aspect of trophoblastic disease was a particular polymorphism of hCG gene seen in choriocarcinoma. We found four polymorphisms at the downstream of the hCG-α gene regarding restriction endonuclease Hind III and EcoR I. We tentatively designated these gametes as R^+H^-, R^+H^+, R^-H^-, and R^-H^+, as shown in Figure 1. The theoretical probability of each gamete was calculated based on the results of the polymorphic distribution [6].

The R^+H^- gamete was the most prevalent in normal placental DNA and hydatidiform mole DNA, showing 71% and 87%, respectively. In contrast, in the case of choriocarcinoma DNA, R^-H^+ gamete was the most prevalent, showing a result of 72%. These observations raise the possibility that a particular DNA arrangement at the hCG-α locus is more susceptible to the development of choriocarcinoma than other arrangements. Possibly this arrangement might relate to the activation of some oncogenes.

Recently we found the expression of the feline sarcoma virus (fms) oncogene in placental tissue. The result of Northern blotting hybridized to fms-complementary DNA showed the expression of fms mRNA in both first- and third-trimester placenta [9]. The fms mRNA levels expressed in the placenta are in amounts sufficient to transform cells to cancer cells in vitro. The levels are almost 100 times more in placenta comparing to that in normal other tissue. In addition to fms, extremely high expression of avian myelocytoma (myc) and mouse osteosarcoma (fos) oncogenes in the human placenta has been reported. At present, the biological significance of highly expressed oncogene in the placenta is still unknown. We assume that these oncogenes are elegantly controlling vigorous proliferation and rapid differentiation of human trophoblasts.

ALTERATION IN STEROID MODULATION OF HCG SYNTHESIS AND SECRETION IN CHORIOCARCINOMA

Despite extensive in vivo and in vitro studies, the factors regulating the production and secretion of hCG have not been well defined. Although several factors such as luteinizing hormone-releasing hormone (LH-RH) and dibutyryl cyclic adenosine monophosphate

(AMP) are known to be involved in the stimulatory regulation of hCG production and secretion [10], factors responsible for the inhibitory regulation remain unclear [19].

Thus, in order to elucidate the inhibitory regulation, the dynamics of production and secretion of hCG were investigated by culturing the tissue explants from normal early placenta and choriocarcinoma in the presence or absence of progesterone. As the regulation of mRNA is one of the crucial steps in controlling protein hormone production, the effect of progesterone on the steady-state cellular levels of hCG-α and hCG-βmRNA was also assessed by the technique of in situ hybridization using labeled cDNA probes corresponding to hCG-α and hCG-β.

In culture of placental explants, progesterone suppressed the secretion of hCG and hCG-α after 48-hour culture in a dose-response manner. The tissue levels of hCG-α and hCG-β also decreased in culture supplemented with progesterone. The in situ hybridization revealed that mean grain count for hCG-α and hCG-βmRNAs in the sections prepared in the presence of progesterone decreased compared with those prepared in the absence of progesterone. The decrease in the mean grain count in progesterone-treated tissue was noted at 24-hour culture and became greater at 144-hour culture. It appears that progesterone inhibits the cellular levels of hCG-α and hCG-βmRNAs, resulting in a decrease in hCG synthesis and secretion in normal placenta.

In contrast with hCG, neither hPL level in the culture medium nor hPL tissue level were decreased by progesterone. Furthermore, the mean grain count for hPLmRNA remained unchanged regardless of the presence or absence of progesterone. These results indicate that progesterone in the same concentrations (5 to 20 μg/mL) that suppressed hCG(α, β)mRNA levels and hCG secretion has no effect on the steady-state cellular level of hPLmRNA and the secretion of hPL. Thus, the inhibitory effect of progesterone

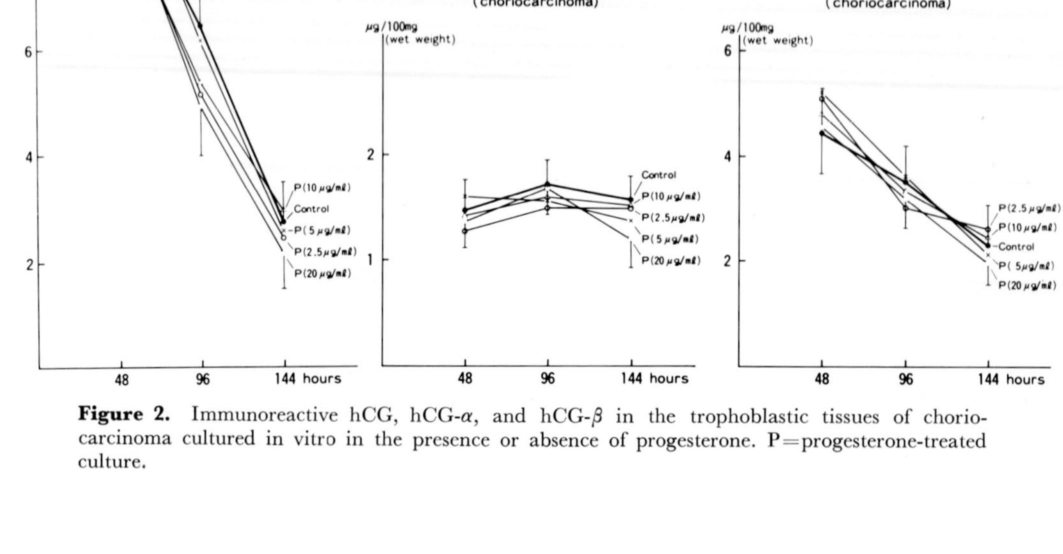

Figure 2. Immunoreactive hCG, hCG-α, and hCG-β in the trophoblastic tissues of choriocarcinoma cultured in vitro in the presence or absence of progesterone. P=progesterone-treated culture.

on hCG(α, β)mRNA levels and hCG secretion does not represent a toxic effect, but rather is a selective effect on hCG synthesis and secretion [11].

On the other hand, in culture of explants of trophoblastic tissues from choriocarcinoma, neither inhibition of the cellular levels of hCG-α and hCG-βmRNAs nor suppression of hCG secretion by progesterone were observed. It is of interest that the tissue levels of hCG and hCG-β drastically declined in the course of culture regardless of the presence or absence of progesterone, whereas the tissue level of hCG-α remained unchanged (Figure 2). These results suggest that hCG newly synthesized in choriocarcinoma more promptly secreted into the culture medium without being accumulated in the cells and that there was no inhibitory regulation of hCG production and secretion by progesterone in choriocarcinoma. Thus, the regulation of hCG synthesis and secretion in choriocarcinoma is different from that in normal placenta [12, 13].

ALTERATION IN STRUCTURE OF SUGAR CHAINS OF HCG PRODUCED BY CHORIOCARCINOMA

Although the biochemical properties of hCG from the urine of normal pregnant women were studied extensively by many investigators, the properties of hCG in patients with choriocarcinoma remained unknown until recently. Thus, we have extracted and purified hCG from the urine of patients with hydatidiform mole and choriocarcinoma, respectively, and analyzed their biochemical properties to compare them with that from normal pregnant women.

Choriocarcinoma hCG showed the same amino acid composition and the same immunoreactivities against anti-hCG, anti-hCG-α, and anti-hCG-β antisera as normal hCG and hydatidiform mole hCG, suggesting that the protein portion of choriocarcinoma hCG is identical to that of normal hCG. However, a great difference in the carbohydrate composition was observed among the three hCG preparations of normal hCG, hydatidiform mole hCG, and choriocarcinoma hCG. Sialic acid content in choriocarcinoma hCG was extremely low or undetectable, whereas normal hCG and hydatidiform mole hCG contained approximately 8.5% sialic acid in the molecule. This result suggested that the malignant transformation of trophoblast may result in an alteration of the glycosylation process, expecially the sialylation of hCG [16].

Thus, in order to elucidate a qualitative alteration of hCG in relation to the malignant transformation of trophoblast, the structure of sugar chains of hCG produced by choriocarcinoma was investigated and compared with that of normal hCG.

Both α- and β-subunits contain two asparagine-linked sugar chains and, in addition, the β-subunit contains four serine-linked sugar chains. In the asparagine-linked sugar chains of normal hCG, all the sialic acid residues were found to occur exclusively as the NeuAcα2→3Gal grouping [1].

The choriocarcinoma hCG was found to possess several prominent structural differences in the sugar chains as compared with normal hCG [14]. More than 97% of the sugar chains of choriocarcinoma hCG was free from sialic acid, whereas the sugar chains of normal hCG were mostly sialylated. Choriocarcinoma hCG contained unusual biantennary complex-type sugar chains in addition to regular tri-, bi-, and monoantennary sugar chains. Furthermore, it was found that occurrence of Galβ1→4GlcNAcβ1→4Manα1→ group is a characteristic feature of the sugar chains of choriocarcinoma hCG, as normal hCG does not contain any triantennary sugar chains. The sum total of fucosylated sugar chains of choriocarcinoma hCG was twice as much as normal hCG, indicating

Table 1. Structural changes in sugar chains of choriocarcinoma hCG

1.	Appearance of sugar chains free from sialic acid
2.	Occurrence of triantennary sugar chains with Galβ1→ 4GlcNAcβ1→4Manα1→ group
3.	Increase in sum total of fucosylated sugar chains

that fucosylation is also modified in choriocarcinoma (Table 1).

In contrast, urinary hCG purified from patients with hydatidiform mole gave almost the same profile of sugar chains as that of normal hCG [1]. It is therefore concluded that the structural changes in the sugar chains of choriocarcinoma hCG observed in our study is specific for malignant transformation of trophoblast.

CLINICAL APPLICATION OF DETECTION OF STRUCTURAL CHANGE OF HCG SUGAR CHAINS FOR THE BIOCHEMICAL DIAGNOSIS OF CHORIOCARCINOMA

Recently we have developed two methods to detect the structural change of sugar chains of choriocarcinoma hCG. One is based on the capability of the lectin from *Arachis hypogala* peanut (PNA) to bind to asialylated sugar chains [18]. The other is an immunological assay method using an antiserum (R141) generated against desialylated hCGβ-COOH-terminal peptide [17].

In PNA-Sepharose affinity chromatography, the entire portion of choriocarcinoma hCG containing no sialic acid was absorbed, whereas the major portion of urinary hCG from normal pregnant women and patients with hydatidiform mole was not absorbed on the column. When the PNA binding of urinary hCG from six patients with choriocarcinoma was studied, two of the six cases (33%) were highly bound to the PNA-Sepharose column. This result suggests that PNA-Sepharose affinity chromatography seems to be an effective means to detect the incompletely sialylated hCG in patients with choriocarcinoma.

On the other hand, in the radioimmunoassay system using the antiserum (R141) generated against enzymatically cleaved, desialylated hCGβ-COOH-terminal peptide, asialo-hCG reacted better than native hCG. With the radioimmunoassay to detect asialo-hCG immunoreactivity, urinary hCG from patients with various trophoblastic diseases were analyzed. The results showed that asialo-hCG immunoreactivity was not found in all patients with hydatidiform mole, invasive mole, and persistent trophoblastic disease examined, whereas urinary hCG from one-third (33%) of patients with choriocarcinoma demonstrated asialo-hCG immunoreactivity. Thus, this immunological method to detect desialylated hCG seems to be a useful means for the biochemical diagnosis of choriocarcinoma.

However, desialylation of sugar chains of hCG does not always appear in patients with choriocarcinoma. Development of a new method to detect the prominent structure of sugar chains of GA1β1→4GlcNAcβ1→4Manα1→ group, which is specific for choriocarcinoma hCG, will be needed to establish the biochemical method to diagnose choriocarcinoma definitely. The development of this new method is now in progress in our laboratory.

ACKNOWLEDGMENT

This work was supported in part by Grant-in-Aid for Scientific Research (No. 60480368, No. 60570776) from the Japanese Ministry of Education, Science, and Culture.

REFERENCES

1. Endo Y, Yamashita K, Tachibana Y, Tojo S, Kobata A: Structures of the asparagine-linked sugar chains of human chorionic gonadotropin. J Biochem 85: 669–679, 1979.
2. Clayton LA, Tyrey L, Weed JC, Hammond CB: Endocrine aspects of trophoblastic neoplasia. J Reprod Med 26: 192–199, 1981.
3. Hoshina M, Ashitaka Y, Tojo S: Immunohistochemical interaction on antisera to hCG and its subunits with chorionic tissue of early gestation. Endocrinol Jpn 26: 175–184, 1979.
4. Hoshina M, Boothby M, Boime I: Cytological localization of chorionic gonadotropin and placental lactogen mRNAs during development of the human placenta. J Cell Biol 93: 190–198, 1982.
5. Hoshina M, Hussa R, Pattillo R, Boime I: Cytological distribution, of chorionic gonadotropin subunit and placental lactogen mRNAs in neoplasma derived from human placenta. J Cell Biol 97: 1200–1206, 1983.
6. Hoshina M, Boothby WR, Hussa RD, Pattillo RA, Camel HM, Boime I: Segregation patterns of polymorphic restriction sites of the hCGα gene in trophoblastic disease. Proc Natl Acad Sci 81: 2504–2507, 1984.
7. Hoshina M, Mochizuki M: The molecular biology of placental protein hormones. ICMR Annals 151–162, 1984.
8. Hoshina M, Hussa R, Pattillo R, Boime I: The role of trophoblast differentiation in the control of the hCG and hPL genes. In Pattillo RA, Hussa RO (eds): Human Trophoblast Neoplasia. Plenum, New York, 1984, pp. 299–313.
9. Hoshina M, Boothby M, Hussa R, Pattillo RA, Camel HM, Boime I: Linkage of human chorionic gonadotropin and placental lactogen biosynthesis to trophoblast differentiation and tumorigenesis: Placenta (in press).
10. Hussa RO: Biosynthesis of human chorionic gonadotropin. Endocr Rev 1: 268–294, 1980.
11. Maruo T, Matsuo H, Otani T, Hoshina M, Mochizuki M: Progesterone-mediated inhibition of chorionic gonadotropin and β-mRNA in trophoblastic tissues cultured in vitro. In Abstracts of 7th International Congress of Endocrinology (International Congress Series 652). Excerpta Medica, New York, 1984, p. 997.
12. Maruo T, Matsuo H, Otani T, Hoshina M, Mochizuki M: Differential modulation of chorionic gonadotropin (CG) subunit messenger ribonucleic acid levels and CG secretion by progesterone in normal placenta and choriocarcinoma cultured in vitro. Endocrinology 119: 1986 (in press).
13. Matsuo H, Maruo T, Hoshina M, Mochizuki M: Selective inhibition of synthesis and secretion of hCG by progesterone and its correlation with hCG (α, β) mRNA levels. Folia Endocrinol 61: 882–892, 1985.
14. Mizuochi T, Nishimura R, Derappe C, Taniguchi T, Hamamoto T, Mochizuki M, Kobata A: Structure of the asparagine-linked sugar chains of human chorionic gonadotropin produced in choriocarcinoma. J Biol Chem 258: 14126–14129, 1983.
15. Mochizuki M, Morikawa H, Kawaguchi K, Tojo S: Growth hormone, prolactin and chorionic somatomammotropin in normal and molar pregnancy. J Clin Endocrinol Metab 43: 614–621, 1976.
16. Nishimura R, Endo Y, Tanabe K, Ashitaka Y, Tojo S: The biochemical properties of urinary human chorionic gonadotropin from the patients with trophoblastic diseases. J Endocrinol Invest 4: 349–358, 1981.
17. Takeuchi Y, Matsuura S, Nishimura R, Mochizuki M: The determination of the recognition site of an antiserum detecting desialylation on O-glycosidic carbohydrates of hCG and its clinical applications. Folia Endocrinol 60: 1046–1057, 1984.
18. Utsunomiya T, Nishimura R, Mochizuki M: Binding of human chorionic gonadotropin with insufficient terminal sugar to peanut aggulutinin. Acta Obstet Gynaecol Jpn 37: 555–561, 1985.
19. Wilson EA, Jawad MJ, Dickson LR: Suppression of human chorionic gonadotropin by progestational steroids. Am J Obstet Gynecol 138: 708–713, 1980.

11

Incidence of Hydatidiform Mole in China: A Preliminary Survey of More than 3 Million Women

Wu Pao-Chen and Song Hong-Zhao

Hydatidiform mole is an unequivocal precursor of malignant gestational trophoblastic diseases, i.e., invasive mole and choriocarcinoma. Invasive mole is almost invariably derived from hydatidiform mole and 69.1% of the patients of choriocarcinoma have a history of molar pregnancy [9]. It is therefore reasonable that any investigation of preventive measures of malignant gestational trophoblastic diseases should begin with a study of the epidemiology of hydatidiform mole. China, as well as many other Asian countries, is known to have a high incidence of hydatidiform mole. However, the incidences reported have been mostly hospital-based and by no means reflect the true status of occurrence of this group of diseases in the general population. The purpose of this report is to present the preliminary results of a retrospective nationwide survey on the incidence of hydatidiform mole in more than 3 million women from prefectures throughout China.

SUBJECTS AND METHOD OF STUDY

To retrospectively investigate the incidence of hydatidiform mole, one must inquire as to the history of past pregnancy in each study subject. This was usually done at the time of a mass screening survey for carcinoma of the cervix, which has been carried out as a routine preventive procedure in some districts of China by local health organizations for many years. In some other units, a special team was organized for this purpose.

After a short study of the feasibility of this investigation by the initiators at the Peking Union Medical College Hospital, the first conference on this subject was held in November 1978 at Shandong Province. At that time a National Collaborative Study Group was founded. The experience obtained from the pilot study and a standardized questionnaire were introduced, together with interviewing requirements. The method of statistical treatment of the data was also formulated.

The formal investigation began in 1979. In addition to direct interviewing of the study subjects, their senior family members were questioned and hospital registration books were checked to remedy possible omissions. Through the collaboration of more than 300 medical centers, hospitals, and women's health care organizations on different levels, a total of 3,089,399 women from 26 provinces, special municipalities, and autonomous regions have been investigated thus far. Approximately 85% of the women were over 30 years of age. Farmers accounted for 70% of the women interviewed, and industrial workers, office workers, teachers, and housewives from urban areas accounted for the remaining 30%. Topographically, the areas investigated covered plains, hilly lands, mountain regions, coastal areas, and islands.

The age and parity of the subjects were documented during inquiry, but were not included in the analysis, because the policy of family planning pursued in the last 20 years may lead to some bias in the interpretation of the data. That is, the advocation of late marriage would certainly have postponed the age of first pregnancy, and restriction of number of siblings in the family would have artificially abolished the occurrence of high parity.

RESULTS

Overall Incidence of Hydatidiform Mole

Among the women surveyed, there was a total of 10,968,218 pregnancies, resulting in 8909 hydatidiform moles. The overall combined incidence was one mole in 1231 pregnancies (0.81‰). The incidences of different provinces are shown in the map in Figure 1. It can be seen that the rates are not too widely scattered, ranging from 0.46 per 1,000 in Shanxi Province to 1.39 per 1000 pregnancies in Chejiang Province.

Geographic Distribution

The figures obtained from different provinces may be divided into three groups—1) an incidence of >1.0 mole per 1,000 pregnancies in five provinces: Chejiang (1.39‰), Guangdong (1.37‰), Hunan (1.14‰), Jiangxi (1.05‰), and Fujian (1.03‰), all situated in the Southeast China and south of the Yangtze River; 2) an incidence of 0.81–1.0 mole per 1,000 pregnancies in eight provinces, municipalities, and autonomous regions, of which four are in the coast area (Shandong, Liaoning, Jiangsu, and Tienjin), two are in the inland region but south of the Yangtze River (Guangxi and Guizhou), and two are purely inland autonomous regions (Xinjiang and Ningxia); 3) an incidence of <0.8 mole per 1000 pregnancies in 13 provinces, municipalities, and autonomous regions, of which 12 are in the inland area and 9 are north of the Yangtze River. The differences between groups 1 and 2, groups 1 and 3, and groups 2 and 3, respectively, are all statistically highly significant ($p<0.001$).

The higher incidence of hydatidiform mole in coastal areas than in inland regions was also demonstrated in some provinces in which a more thorough investigation was carried out for different prefectures. For instance, in Hebei Province the incidence in Tangshan, a seaside prefecture, was 1.02 per 1000 pregnancies (147 moles in 144,011 pregnancies). In contrast, five inland prefectures— Shijiazhuang, Baoding, Langfang, Chengde, and Zhangjiakou—had incidences of 0.61, 0.50, 0.54, 0.69, and 0.62 per 1,000 pregnancies, respectively (Figure 2). The difference between the incidence of Tangshan

PART FOUR

MANAGEMENT OF TROPHOBLASTIC DISEASES

12

Approach for Attaining Complete Cure of Trophoblastic Disease

Yutaka Tomoda, Shigeaki Kaseki, Setsuko Goto, Takao Ishizuka, Yoshihito Furuhashi, Sachihito Katoh, and Hisao Mano

INTRODUCTION

Recent advances in the intensive care system have improved therapeutic results of choriocarcinoma treatment. Invasive mole is now favorably treated with a remission rate of approximately 100%; however, some choriocarcinoma patients still die.

With the goal of finding some treatment that will help attain complete cure of trophoblastic disease, we present a clinical analysis of 549 patients with gestational trophoblastic disease.

MATERIALS AND METHODS

During a period of 28 years from 1957 through 1984, a total of 549 patients with gestational trophoblastic disease were treated at the Department of Obstetrics and Gynecology, School of Medicine, Nagoya University, Nagoya, Japan. There were 186 cases of choriocarcinoma and 363 cases of invasive mole. The 36 cases of choriocarcinoma and 210 cases of invasive mole were given clinical diagnoses based on the choriocarcinoma risk score table devised by Ishizuka [4].

Based on improvements in treatment, the 28 years from 1957 through 1984 were divided into four periods. In the first period, patients were treated by nitrogen mustard, mytomycin-C, and methotrexate (MTX). In thc second period, a single administration of actinomycin-D (act-D) was utilized. In the third period, the combined administration of MTX and act-D was used and surgical intervention for pulmonary metastases was adopted. The fourth period was the time of so-called multidisciplinary treatment, including whole-brain irradiation and immunotherapy.

Table 1 shows the change of diagnostic criteria of complete remission accompanied by improvement in methods of human chorionic gonadotropin (hCG) determination. Based on improvement in the methods of hCG determination, the 28 years were divided into four periods: in the first period, Friedmann's reaction and hemoagglutination inhibition reaction were used; in the second period, an anti-hCG radioimmunoassay system was used; and in the third and fourth periods, an anti-hCG-β radioimmunoassay system was used.

RESULTS

Mortality of Trophoblastic Disease

Figure 1 shows the time trend of mortality of patients with trophoblastic disease by 3-year moving averages. The mortality was 45.5% in 1960. It gradually decreased year by year, and dropped remarkably to 2.2% in 1983. These favorable results were due to recent progress in the diagnosis and treatment of trophoblastic disease.

The time trend of treatment results of gestational trophoblastic disease in relation to metastatic cases and nonmetastatic cases is shown in Figure 2. The mortality of metastatic

Table 1. Criteria of complete remission from trophoblastic disease

Period	Assay method	hCG value
1957–1968	Friedmann's reaction, HAIR	<50 RU (Rabbit unit) in urine, <1 IU/mL in urine
1969–Aug. 1973	hCG RIA	<20 IU/day in urine, LH peak (+)
Sept. 1973–1983	hCG-β RIA	<16 mIU/mL in urine, <5 mIU/mL in serum, no cellular response in the last 2 chemotherpay courses
1984–	hCG-β RIA	<5 mIU/mL in serum, no cellular response in the last 5 chemotherapy courses

HAIR=hemoagglutination inhibition reaction; hCG=human chorionic gonadotropin; hCG-β RIA=anti-hCG-β radioimmunoassay; hCG RIA=anti-hCG radioimmunoassay; LH=luteinizing hormone.

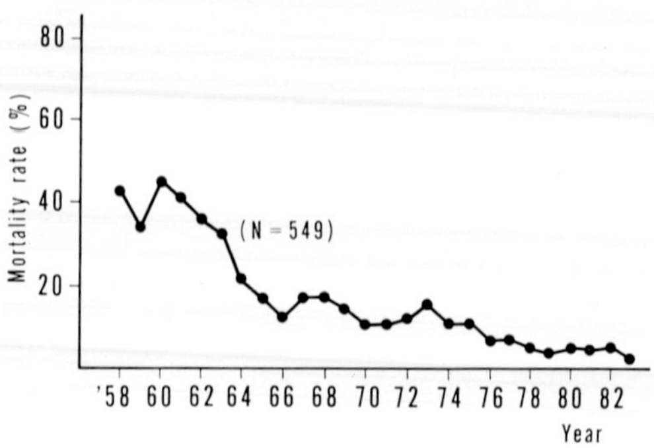

Figure 1. Results of treatment for trophoblastic disease.

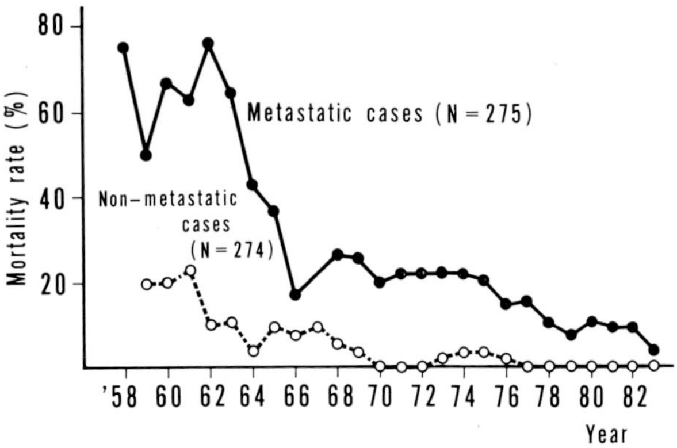

Figure 2. Results of treatment for metastatic and nonmetastatic cases.

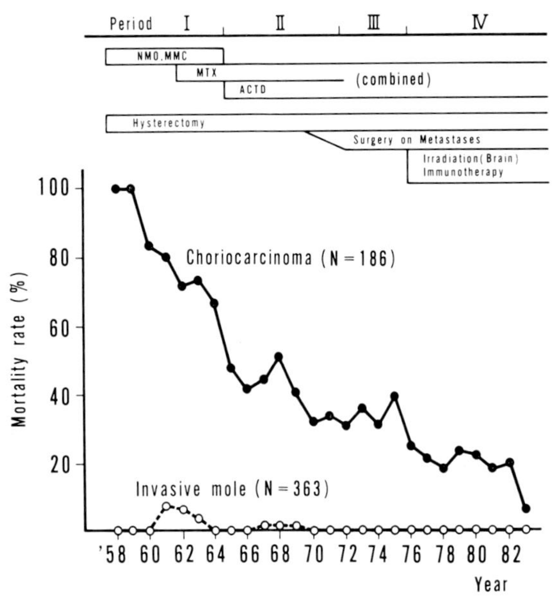

Figure 3. Results of treatment for invasive mole and choriocarcinoma.

cases dropped remarkably through the use of combined administration of MTX with act-D, and the gradual decrease continued thereafter. The mortality of nonmetastatic cases reached 0% in 1977.

The treatment results of gestational trophoblastic disease in relation to invasive moles and choriocarcinomas are illustrated in Figure 3. The mortality of invasive moles was 0% continuously since 1970. On the other hand, the mortality of choriocarcinomas, which was 100% in 1958, gradually decreased and finally dropped to 6.7% in 1983.

The above-mentioned results indicate that complete cure of gestational trophoblastic disease means that the mortality of choriocarcinoma reaches 0%. When the treatment results were compared between metastatic cases and nonmetastatic cases in choriocarcinoma, the mortality, which decreased in both groups over time, had already reached 0% in nonmetastatic cases, but it still was about 20% in metastatic cases (Figure 4). These

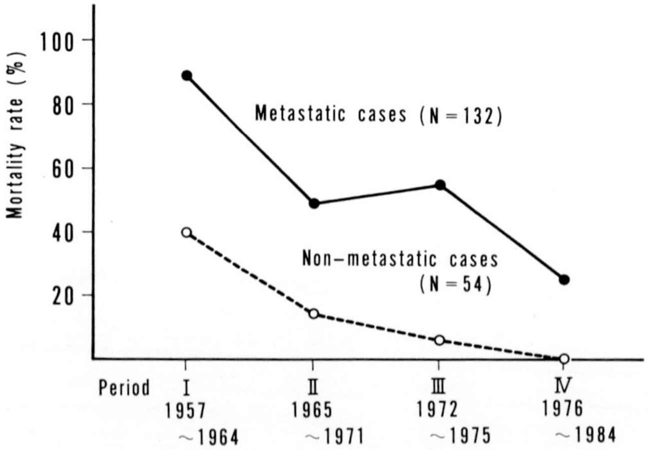

Figure 4. Results of treatment for metastatic and nonmetastatic choriocarcinoma.

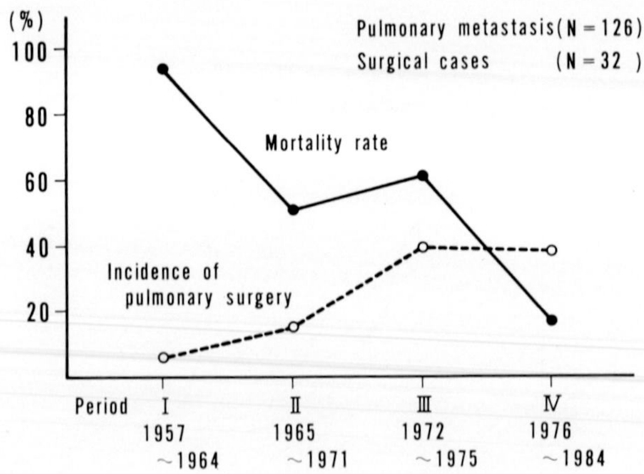

Figure 5. Mortality and incidence of surgery for pulmonary metastases of choriocarcinoma.

facts made it clear that the most important subject for study is how to treat the metastatic focus of choriocarcinoma.

Surgical Treatment for Pulmonary Metastases

Figure 5 exhibits the relationship between the incidence of performing thoracotomy and the mortality in choriocarcinoma patients with pulmonary metastases. With the increase of pulmonary surgery, the mortality decreased. After 1972, about 40% of patients with pulmonary metastases received thoracotomy and the mortality remarkably decreased. The effect of surgery was clearly proved.

Figure 6 shows the alteration of hCG values in choriocarcinoma patients with pulmonary metastases. The darkened area indicates the hCG values in patients cured by chemotherapy alone. As shown in this figure, in patients whose hCG values do not become negative within 10 weeks after dropping below 1,000 mIU/mL, the hCG value gradually reelevates and the patient dies. Therefore, it is very difficult for patients whose hCG values are still positive at 10 weeks after dropping below 1,000 mIU/mL to attain

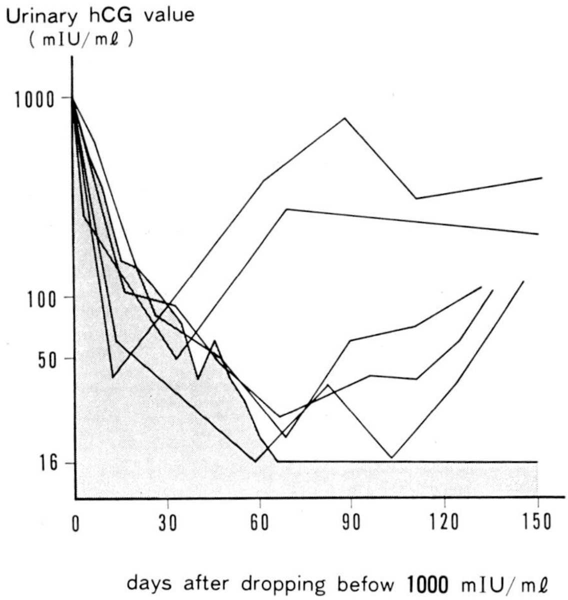

Figure 6. Alteration of hCG values in patients that died of pulmonary metastases of choriocarcinoma (nonsurgical cases).

Table 2. Conditions for achieving good results by thoracotomy for pulmonary metastases of choriocarcinoma

1. In patients whose urinary hCG values have been below 1,000 mIU/mL for over 10 weeks, these values must still be detectable.
2. Patients must be at good risk for surgical intervention.
3. There must be no evidence of primary or metastatic foci elsewhere in the body.
4. The metastases must be resectable by one operation.

Table 3. Results of surgical treatment for pulmonary metastases of choriocarcinoma

Meeting of four conditions	No. of cases	Complete remission
Satisfactory	20	100%
Unsatisfactory	12	33%*

* Relapse and death in four cases.

complete remission by chemotherapy alone, and it is optimal at that time to undertake surgical intervention.

Four conditions for achieving good results by pulmonary surgery are listed in Table 2. Table 3 shows the results of treatment in patients receiving thoracotomy in relation to satisfaction of these four conditions. The rate of complete remission in the patients who satisfied the four conditions was 100%. However, the remission rate was only 33% in those who did not satisfy them.

Treatment for Intracranial Metastases

Figure 7 illustrates the prognosis of choriocarcinoma patients with intracranial metastases

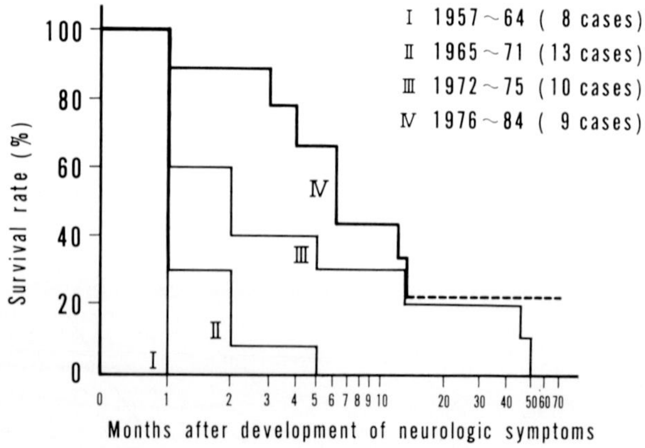

Figure 7. Survival curve for intracranial metastases of choriocarcinoma.

Table 4. Analysis of intracranial metastatic foci (30 autopsy cases)

No. of foci	No. of cases
Solitary	18 (60%)
Multiple	12 (40%)

Site and depth	No. of foci
Cerebrum	43 (91.4%)
Superficial	22 (46.8%)
Intermediate	16 (34.0%)
Deep	5 (10.6%)
Cerebellum	4 (8.5%)

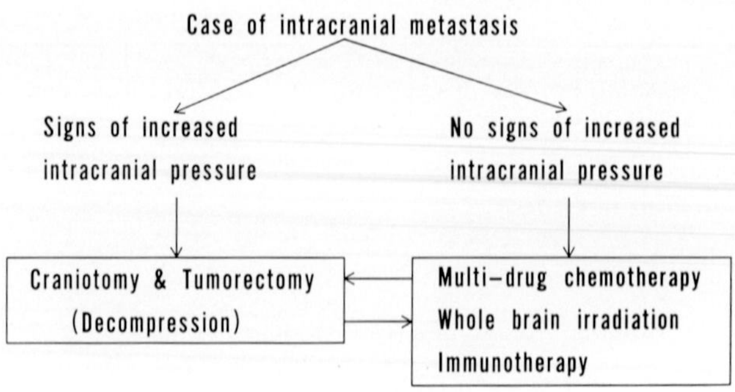

Figure 8. Treatment for intracranial metastases.

in relation to the period by the Kaplan-Meier's life-table method. The survival time was elongated over time, and in the fourth period, when the craniotomy and whole-brain irradiation were positively undertaken, complete remission and cure was experienced in several cases.

Table 4 demonstrates the condition of intracranial metastatic foci of choriocarcinoma by postmortem analysis. As to the number, the solitary focus was seen in 60%. The findings obtained from studies of the site, depth, and number of metastatic foci suggest that metastatic intracranial foci can be removed surgically in most patients.

Figure 8 outlines the treatment modality for the patients with intracranial metastases [5]. If signs of increased intracranial pressure are present, removal of the tumor, or at least decompression, should be immediately performed to save the patient from the immediate danger. If these symptoms are not present, chemotherapy combined with irradiation is the first treatment of choice.

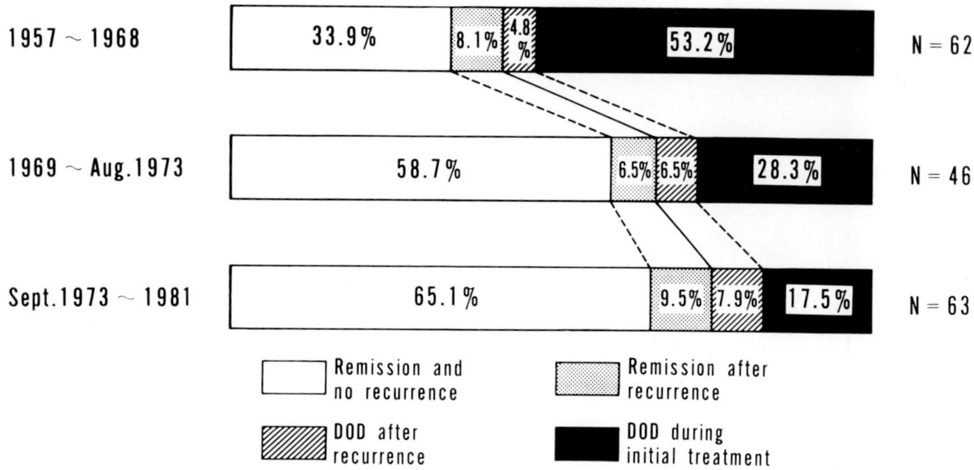

Figure 9. Analysis of treatment results for choriocarcinoma. DOD=dead of disease.

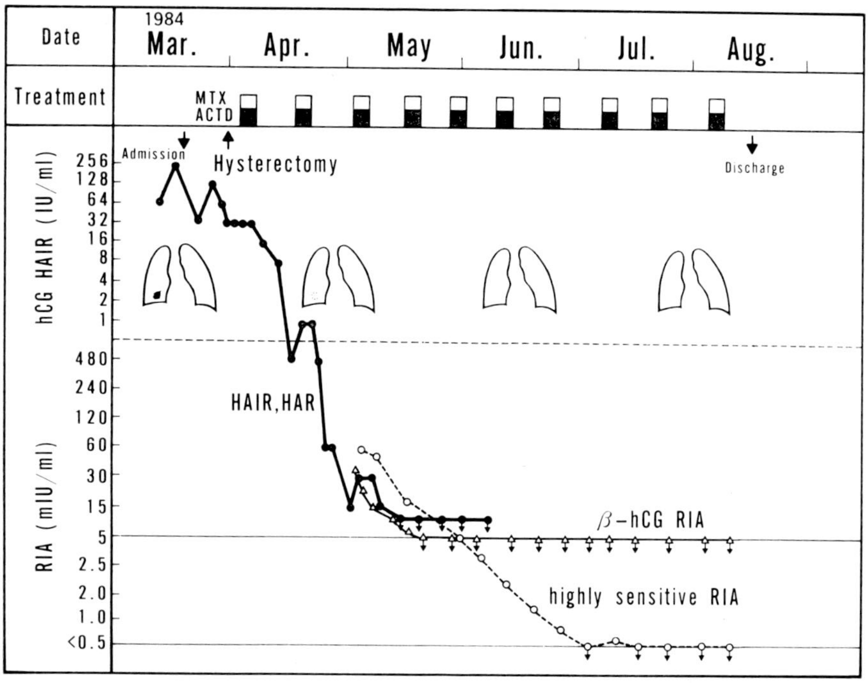

Figure 10. hCG pattern in a patient with choriocarcinoma.

Recurrence in Patients with Choriocarcinoma

Figure 9 displays the results of treatment of choriocarcinoma in relation to the three periods. Comparison among the three periods reveals that the number of the patients who attained complete remission without later recurrence increased since 1973, and the number of patients that died during the first treatment remarkably decreased. However, the number of patients that died after recurrence did not decrease.

Therefore, the prevention of recurrence and death should be the first step for obtaining favorable results in a decrease of mortality in choriocarcinoma [3].

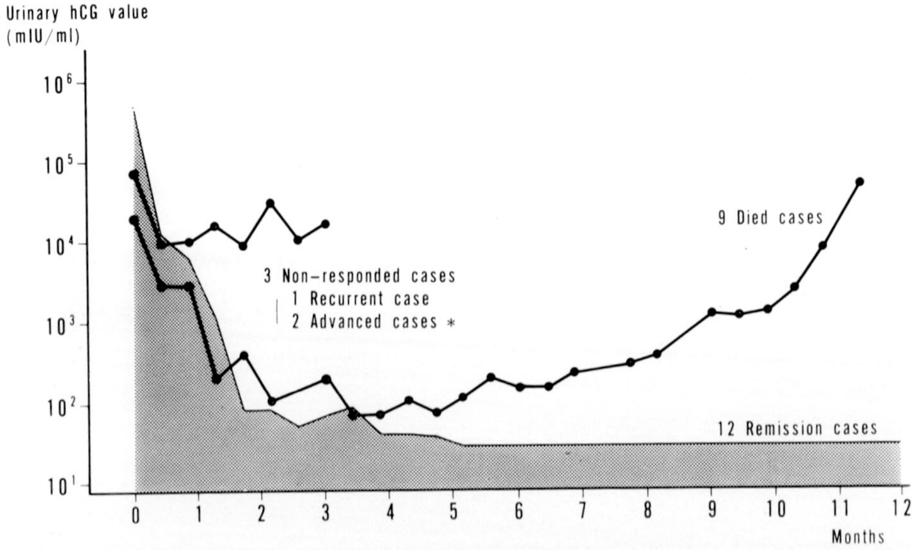

Figure 11. Alterations in mean hCG values in patients that died.

Figure 10 shows alteration of hCG values in a choriocarcinoma patient, as determined by anti-hCG-β radioimmunoassay and highly sensitive radioimmunoassay developed by our laboratory [6].

After hCG value was less than 5 mIU/mL, as determined by anti-hCG-β radioimmunoassay, hCG value was still detectable by the highly sensitive assay. The hCG value gradually decreased to below 0.5 mIU/mL.

Therefore, a larger number of chemotherapeutic courses, more than used in the past, was thought necessary [13]. These results may indicate that at least five to six additional chemotherapeutic courses should be given after hCG value drops below 5 mIU/mL.

Clinical Courses of Patients that Died

Alterations in mean hCG values in three groups of choriocarcinoma patients treated after 1957 are shown in Figure 11. The three nonresponding cases consisted of one patient treated after recurrence and two patients who were initially treated at other hospitals.

The hCG values of 21 cases responding to treatment reached a low level in the period from 3 to 5 months after the initiation of treatment. This period was considered critical. The hCG values in 12 remission cases continued to be negative, whereas the values re-elevated in nine patients that died after this period.

As this period is most important for the treatment of choriocarcinoma, new methods of treatment and diagnosis should be introduced. Possible examples might include new chemotherapeutic agents, biological-response modifiers, and new techniques for detection of the fine foci that cannot be found by the usual methods.

In this critical period, the foci became unclear in 6 of 12 patients that died. Had these fine foci been clarified, proper measures could have been taken.

DISCUSSION

Treatment results for patients with choriocarcinoma at different hospitals have been reported. Lurain et al. [7] stated that 129 of 159 patients (81%) with choriocarcinoma were cured at the Brewer Trophoblastic Disease Center of Northwestern University Medical School from 1962 through 1978. Survit et al. [11] documented that nine of the ten patients with poor-prognosis gestational trophoblastic neoplasia treated at Southwestern Regional Trophoblastic Disease Center from 1979 to 1983 were in complete remission for 4 to 44 months. According to Newland and Bagshawe [9], the mortality of patients with choriocarcinoma was 5.6% (3/54) in 1979 to 1981 at Charing Cross Hospital. According to reports from other hospitals in Japan [8, 12], the mortality of patients with choriocarcinoma was about 40%. It is suggested that the diagnostic standard of choriocarcinoma may be different in Japan than in other countries. The present authors showed that the mortality of patients with choriocarcinoma gradually decreased and finally dropped to 6.7% in 1983. These favorable results were partially brought about by surgery for pulmonary and intracranial metastatic foci.

Few treatment results of pulmonary surgery have been reported. According to Hammond et al. [2] thoracotomy was performed in 11 patients, 4 of whom were in remission. In the present study, 20 of 32 patients undergoing lung operations achieved remission. Surgical indications for resection in pulmonary metastases have already been proposed [14], and results of the present study emphasize the significance of timing of surgical procedures.

Weed and Hammond [15] reported that 50% of 14 patients with brain metastases of choriocarcinoma obtained remission after vigorous, multiagent chemotherapy and combined cerebral irradiation therapy. Craniotomy was performed in 5 of the 14 patients. According to Athanassiou et al. [1], 18 of 69 patients with central nervous system metastases were in remission, and five of seven patients with cerebral operation were alive and off treatment. The findings of depth and number of metastatic foci obtained from the present study suggest that metastatic intracranial foci could be removed surgically in most patients.

Analysis of the cases in which the patient died suggests that changes of chemotherapeutic regimen were not effective in resistant cases. Therefore, biological-response modifiers and new techniques for detection of the fine foci should be introduced. The present authors are now considering clinical application of radioimmunodetection method by monoclonal antibody against placental alkaline phosphatase.

There are a few reports about recurrence of trophoblastic disease. Survit et al. [10] stated that 11 patients (26%) in the poor-prognosis category developed recurrences after achieving primary remission, and the mortality of patients with recurrent gestational trophoblastic neoplasia with high-risk disease was 63.6% (7/11). Takamizawa et al. [12] demonstrated that the recurrent rate of choriocarcinoma was 28.6% (6/21) and that four of six patients with recurrence died. In the present study, the recurrence rate of choriocarcinoma and the mortality of patients with recurrence were 21.9% (25/114) and 44.0% (11/25), respectively. Prevention of the recurrence is an important issue to be considered. The application of newer diagnostic criteria for complete remission and undertaking a trial study of maintenance therapy for cases with a high risk of recurrence should be considered.

The present authors are attempting to achieve 100% cure of choriocarcinoma, a final goal that is near.

REFERENCES

1. Athanassiou A, Begent RHJ, Newland ES et al.: Central nervous system metastases of choriocarcinoma: 23 years' experience at Charing Cross Hospital. Cancer 52: 1728–1735, 1983.
2. Hammond CB, Weed JC, Currie JL, et al.: The role of operation in the current therapy of gestational trophoblastic disease. Am J Obstet Gynecol 136: 844–858, 1980.
3. Hirokawa K, Tomoda Y, Kaseki S, et al.: Recurrence of invasive moles and choriocarcinomas. Asia-Oceania J Obstet Gynecol 18: 11–20, 1986.
4. Ishizuka N: Studies on trophoblastic neoplasia. In: Cancer in Asia (Gann Monograph on Cancer Research, vol. 18). University of Tokyo Press, Tokyo, 1976, pp. 203–216.
5. Ishizuka T, Tomoda Y, Kaseki S, et al.: Intracranial metastasis of choriocarcinoma: A clinicopathologic study. Cancer 52: 1896–1903, 1983.
6. Katoh S, Hattori S, Furuhashi Y, et al.: Highly sensitive, competitive radio-immunoassay for human chorionic gonadtropin extracted from serum by a solid phase monoclonal antibody. Endocrinol Japan (in press).
7. Lurain JR, Brewer JI, Torok EE, et al.: Gestational trophoblastic disease: Treatment results at the Brewer Trophoblastic Center. Obstet Gynecol 60: 354–360, 1982.
8. Mochizuki M, Ashitaka Y, Maruo T, et al.: Sixteen years experience in treatment and follow-up of patients with trophoblastic disease. Asia-Oceania J Obstet Gynecol 10: 15–24, 1984.
9. Newland ES, Bagshawe KD: The role of VP-213 (Etoposide; NSC-141540) in gestational choriocarcinoma. Cancer Chemother Pharmacol 7: 211–214, 1982.
10. Survit EA, Hammond CB: Recurrent gestational trophoblastic disease. Gynecol Oncol 12: 177–185, 1981.
11. Survit EA, Alberts DS, Chris CD, et al.: Poor-prognosis gestational trophoblastic disease: An update. Obstet Gynecol 64: 21–26, 1984.
12. Takamizawa Y, Kobayashi O, Katoh T, et al.: Studies on the recurrence of trophoblastic disease. Acta Obstet Gynaecol Jpn 34: 1729–1735, 1982.
13. Tomoda Y, Asai Y, Arii Y, et al.: Criteria of complete remission from trophoblastic neoplasia with the use of human chorionic gonadtropin excretion pattern as a parameter. Cancer 40: 1016–1025, 1977.
14. Tomoda Y, Arii Y, Kaseki S, et al.: Surgical indication for resection in pulmonary metastasis of choriocarcinoma. Cancer 46: 2723–2730, 1980.
15. Weed JC, Hammond CB: Cerebral metastatic choriocarcinoma: Intensitive therapy and prognosis. Obstet Gynecol 55: 89–94, 1980.

13

Clinical Management and Neoplastic Sequelae of Trophoblastic Embolization Associated with Hydatidiform Mole

Ernest I. Kohorn

Embolization of hydatidiform molar tissue to the pulmonary vasculature is the one remaining potentially life-threatening complication of hydatidiform mole. The previously frequent complications of hemorrhage and infection should become rare with the available sophisticated means of early diagnosis of hydatidiform molar pregnancy [18] and subsequent immediate evacuation. However, molar embolization may present early in the first trimester and may then be the presenting clinical condition or, more usually, may become clinically evident at the time of or soon after mole evacuation.

Embolization of trophoblast in hydatidiform mole was first reported by Trotter and Tieche [19] and by Lipp et al. [14], who documented the presence of villous trophoblast in the pulmonary vasculature at postmortem examination. Recently Twiggs [21] demonstrated syncytiotrophoblast and trophoblastic giant cells in samples of pulmonary arterial blood obtained by means of a Swan-Ganz catheter during successful cardiac monitering of a patient with embolization. The pathophysiology of the condition is therefore beyond doubt, although the differentiation from other causes of cardiopulmonary distress may occasionally still be difficult [21]. This syndrome of hydatidiform mole embolization differs in time of clinical presentation from the various pulmonary manifestations of trophoblastic neoplasia described by Bagshawe [1]. Recognition of the subclinical condition and management of the syndrome have been described in several reports [12, 16, 20]. However, measurement of arterial oxygen tension as an aid in the diagnosis of the patient at risk for embolization is still not practiced routinely, and the use of high-dose steroids in management remains debatable. This paper discusses the diagnosis and management of molar embolization and the frequency of postembolization trophoblastic neoplasia.

DIFFERENTIAL DIAGNOSIS

Until recently there has been difficulty and even controversy in distinguishing between molar deportation and other pulmonary complications of hydatidiform mole [6, 8, 11]. These complications include congestive cardiac failure associated with 1) excess of thyrotropic-like hormone; 2) pulmonary congestion associated with severe anemia following chronic blood loss from the uterus, possibly aggravated by deficient iron intake; and 3) pulmonary changes from fluid overload following overzealous infusion of fluid when the patient was not fluid depleted. One or more of these factors may coexist.

Thyrotoxicosis

A moderately elevated level of thyroid hormone is frequently found particularly with more mature molar pregnancy [9, 10] associated with a high human chorionic gonadotropin (hCG) level. Although there may be tachycardia and even tremor, gross clinical thyrotoxicosis is uncommon [17]. It is rarely a problem if the mole is treated early.

Thyrotoxicosis leading to congestive cardiac failure is unusual. Twiggs [21] recently reviewed the significance of the hyperthyroid syndrome with hydatidiform mole. It rarely becomes necessary to administer sodium iodide or to use propranolol to induce a beta blockade to lessen the cardiac effects of the thyrotoxicosis. It is agreed that the treatment of hydatidiform mole associated thyrotoxicosis is immediate evacuation of the mole and this will nearly invariably lead to spontaneous resolution of the hyperthyroid state. If there is postevacuation persistence of thyrotoxicosis, more detailed evaluation may be indicated.

ANEMIA AND HYPERVOLEMIA

Pritchard [17], using ^{59}Fe blood and red cell studies in patients with hydatidiform mole, concluded that five of eight patients had a significantly increased blood volume with relative anemia. Cotton et al. [4] monitored seven patients with hydatidiform mole who had a significantly enlarged uterus by means of a Swan-Ganz catheter before, during, and after mole evacuation. None of these patients had pulmonary symptoms, but all showed mild transient depression of ventricular performance with recovery after anesthesia. The mean plasma volume in these patients was not increased.

FLUID ADMINISTRATION AND CORRECTION OF ANEMIA DURING MANAGEMENT OF MOLAR PREGNANCY

In reviewing reports of pulmonary complications during therapy for hydatidiform mole, it appears that a significant part of the problem is frequently associated with iatrogenic fluid overload. The scenario goes something like this: An anemic patient whose blood volume has in fact corrected itself following repeated small episodes of bleeding into the uterus is transfused with whole blood. The patient may indeed require transfusion with packed cells to replenish red cell mass before regional or general anesthesia for mole evacuation. Then at the time of suction curettage, a dramatic volume of blood is evacuated from the uterus. This is "old blood," the volume of which, though substantial, has long been replaced in the vascular compartment. No transfusion is indicated. But because of the dramatic "hemorrhage," more blood is now given. Soon after this, the patient develops congestive cardiac failure, which is attributed to the clinical condition of hydatidiform mole.

It is evident that if a patient presents with anemia, blood replacement should be done by transfusion of packed red cells. If fluid is administered in any significant volume, this should be done by careful monitoring of central venous pressure. Use of a Swan-Ganz catheter is preferred in patients undergoing high-risk cardiac monitoring.

OTHER PULMONARY PATHOLOGIC STATES

Chronic pulmonary disease, heart disease, and essential hypertension are unusual in patients with hydatidiform mole. If present, there is usually a history of these conditions. Preeclamptic toxemia may complicate the management of the cardiopulmonary complications of molar pregnancy patients.

INCIDENCE OF TROPHOBLASTIC EMBOLIZATION IN PATIENTS WITH HYDATIDIFORM MOLE

Among 189 patients with hydatidiform mole at Yale Medical Center from 1971 to 1983, pulmonary embolization occurred five times (2.6%). Of these patients, 45 had a uterus that was 4 weeks or more larger than gestational age, giving an incidence of 11% for this high-risk group. Among 306 patients managed at the New England Trophoblastic Disease Center, six patients developed this syndrome (1.9%) [12]. Twiggs et al. [20] reported 128 patients with mole. Of these patients, 44 had a uterus larger than 16 weeks gestational size, and 12 developed respiratory complications, including seven definite embolizations. The rate of embolization among the 128 patients was thus 5.4%, and it was 15.9% in the group with a large uterus. The report of Morrow et al. [15], from the same center, indicated that in their patient population a high proportion of moles presented late, and this may explain the high frequency of pulmonary complications in the report by Twiggs et al.

CLINICAL PRESENTATION

The presentation of molar embolization may be subclinical or manifest. If the patient presents with symptoms of pulmonary distress (Figure 1), it is important that an associated pregnancy is recognized as a molar pregnancy. Ultrasound examination should settle this matter speedily. One of two patients with severe embolization reported here was treated for "pneumonia" for a week before the pregnancy was recognized, the mole diagnosed, and the correct diagnosis made. In such patients with clinically evident pulmonary insufficiency, invasive cardiac monitoring and serial blood gas measurement should be instituted at once and continued until the patient's condition is stable.

With milder cases of embolization, symptoms may be absent or minimal. One of our earlier cases was a patient whose only symptom was her insistence on sitting up and her refusal to lie down. Results of clinical examination and chest x-rays before evacuation

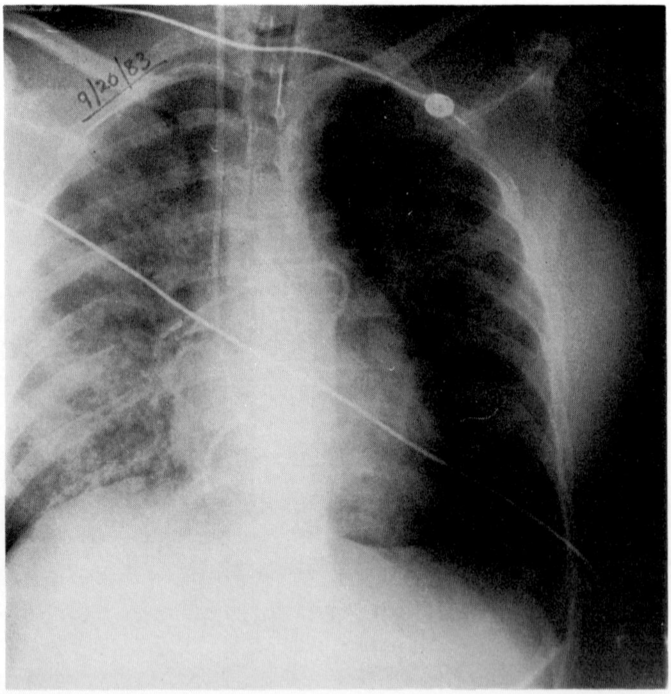

Figure 1. Lungs in a patient with a hydatidiform mole of 20-week uterine size at 8 weeks' gestational age after therapy for "pneumonia" for 7 days before diagnosis of the gestation. Following mole evacuation with invasive cardiac monitoring, mechanical ventilation was necessary for 48 hours (positive end expiratory pressure, 10 to 15 cm/H_2O). The pulmonary status improved and the lungs cleared after 4 days. Chemotherapy was later necessary for nonmetastatic gestational trophoblastic neoplasia.

were abnormal, and only after her condition deteriorated after mole evacuation were infiltrates seen on the chest x-ray. Lung scan findings were also abnormal after mole evacuation.

It is generally agreed that the patient at risk is the one whose uterus is 4 weeks or more larger than gestational age, and particularly a uterus larger than 16 to 20 weeks' gestational size [12, 16, 20]. Frequently, a careful history taking will elicit mild pulmonary symptoms, but more usually the arterial oxygen tension will be reduced in those patients, who are likely to develop clinically threatening pulmonary insufficiency during or shortly after evacuation. All patients who fall into this risk group of an enlarged uterus for dates should have arterial gas estimations on admission. If the arterial gas values are normal, routine monitoring is employed, but no central line is placed, unless there are other indications such as severe anemia or blood loss. If the arterial gas values, particularly the oxygen tension, are reduced, then we consider Swan-Ganz cardiac monitoring advisable during and immediately after mole evacuation.

MANAGEMENT

All reports on trophoblastic embolization of molar tissue agree that evacuation of the mole as soon as the patient's condition has been stabilized is mandatory. Once this is accomplished, the disease is self-limiting. If indicated, oxygen should be administered by the nasal route, by mask, or by intubation, with mechanical ventilation if necessary. Anemia is corrected by transfusion of packed red cells, not whole blood. Fluid administration and the use of diuretics may be monitored by the use of invasive cardiac monitoring [2, 4]. A central venous line is an essential minimal necessity, but measurement of central venous pressure, pulmonary arterial pressure, and pulmonary wedge pressure will give a more precise assessment, particularly when combined with blood gas estimations and measurement of blood volume. Such techniques are now available in all centers practicing cardiac surgery, and directors of trophoblast centers should develop a protocol with their departments of anesthesia, pulmonary medicine, and cardiology for the management of such patients. Whenever possible, a patient with mole who is at high risk for embolization should be treated at a trophoblast center or at least in a hospital with facilities for sophisticated cardiopulmonary monitoring.

We have found the use of general anesthesia easier for the patient, as intubation and positive pressure respiration are thus more easily tolerated. However, in mild cases regional anesthesia may be used, whereas in very ill patients pudendal and paracervical block may be indicated. Because a contracted uterus allows for safer curettage and occludes the myometrial veins, perhaps preventing further embolization during the surgical procedure, oxytocin (Syntocinon) infusion, 40 U/liter, is commenced as the cervix is being dilated. Once the bulk of the mole has been evacuated, methylergonovine maleate (Methergine) or ergometrine is given if the uterus does not contract well, provided there is no hypertension. Cardiopulmonary monitoring and positive pressure respiration using a mechanical ventilator are continued as long as necessary following mole evacuation.

Besides good sedation, oxygen administration, appropriate mechanical ventilation, careful invasive cardiopulmonary monitoring of fluid and blood administration, and mole evacuation, steroids in high dose should be administered as soon as the diagnosis of embolization is established. The pulmonary edema and alveolar exudate appear to be secondary to the foreign protein present. In one patient in the present series who had postpartum preeclampsia, steroids were withheld for 36 hours, with no improvement of pulmonary status. Once methylprednisolone sodium succinate (Solu-Medrol) was given, there was dramatic improvement, with no aggravation of the hypertension. With the patient who died, reported by Orr et al. [16], steroids were not administered until the third day of management. The reported experience with steroids so far is limited [12] and even anecdotal. However, the use of a short course of high-dose steroids has not been associated with any complication, and there has been dramatic clinical improvement in pulmonary function with resolution of pulmonary exudate. This therapy is strongly advocated.

It is noteworthy that the pulmonary status of these patients and the radiologic appearance of the chest improves speedily, probably much more so than with pulmonary embolus.

TROPHOBLASTIC SEQUELAE

Morrow et al. [15] and then Orr et al. [16] drew attention to the high frequency of trophoblastic neoplasia following pulmonary embolization of molar tissue. However, few reports of hydatidiform mole give data that correlate pulmonary embolization with the incidence of subsequent trophoblastic neoplasia. Orr et al. [16] reported eight patients with embolization, one of whom died. The remaining seven patients all required chemotherapy for persistently elevated hCG titers. None developed metastases.

Twiggs et al. [20] reported that 12 of 128 patients with hydatidiform mole had "acute severe respiratory embarassment" during hospitalization. In all cases the onset

Table 1. Neoplastic sequelae of trophoblastic embolization with hydatidiform mole

Total no. of moles	No. of embolizations (%)	Neoplastic sequelae following embolization	Author
128	7 (5.4)	7	Twiggs et al.
189	5 (2.6)	5*	Kohorn
230	8 (3.4)†	7	Orr et al.

* One patient received prophylactic chemotherapy.
† One patient died of adult respiratory distress.

of symptoms was within 12 hours of evacuation. None of these patients required ventilatory assistance, and all blood gas values reverted to normal within 72 hours of evacuation. Twiggs et al. concluded that 7 of the 12 patients had trophoblastic embolization, and that of the remaining five patients, one had thyrotoxicosis, one had obvious iatrogenic fluid overload, and the etiology in the remaining three patients was uncertain. The seven patients with definite embolization required chemotherapy for nonmetastatic neoplasia.

In the present Yale series, all five patients with embolization required subsequent chemotherapy; none developed lung metastases. In fact, one of our patients received prophylactic actinomycin-D immediately after recovery from the acute respiratory state, yet her hCG level remained elevated and she required two further courses of actinomycin-D to achieve remission.

The use of prophylactic chemotherapy has been shown to prevent the development of metastases and to reduce significantly the incidence of nonmetastatic neoplasia [7]. Prophylactic chemotherapy clearly has a definite place in the treatment of patients who may not be followed up with certainty. It has not found general acceptance in populations in which patients may be followed assiduously by serial weekly hCG titer measurements [13]. This is because the remission rate among patients who are followed up closely and who are treated with chemotherapy as soon as they develop persistently elevated hCG titers is virtually 100%. Patients with mole who have a high hCG titer, an enlarged uterus for dates, and theca-lutein cysts have been identified as a group at higher risk for trophoblastic sequelae [5]. Berkowitz and Goldstein [3] have suggested that this group of mole patients should be given prophylactic chemotherapy. However, even by their criteria the risk of neoplasia is only 50%, and if the patient can be followed up reliably it would seem preferable to give chemotherapy only when indicated by hCG evaluation. Patients with pulmonary embolization of mole appear to have a virtual 100% chance of developing nonmetastatic trophoblastic neoplasia (Table 1). This therefore appears to be the group to whom chemotherapy should be given once the acute pulmonary episode has resolved. This chemotherapy needs to be adjuvant rather than prophylactic in the sense that courses will need to be continued until the hCG level becomes undetectable.

ACKNOWLEDGMENT

This paper is reprinted from The Obstetrical and Gynecological Survey with full permission of the editors.

REFERENCES

1. Bagshawe KD: Choriocarcinoma: The Clinical Biology of the Trophoblast and Its Tumors. Williams & Wilkins, Baltimore, 1969, pp. 45–46 and 93–103.

2. Benedetti TJ, Twiggs LB, Morrow CP: Pre- and postevacuation hemodynamic and metabolic studies of hydatidiform mole and severe pregnancy-induced hypertension: A case report. J Reprod Med 25: 133–134, 1980.
3. Berkowitz RS, Goldstein DP: The diagnosis and management of molar pregnancy. In Gestational Trophoblastic Neoplasms (Major Problems in Obstetrics and Gynecology, vol. 14). Saunders, Philadelphia, 1982, pp. 168–170.
4. Cotton DB, Bernstein SG, Read JA, Benedetti TJ, D'Ablaing G, Miller FC, Morrow CP: Hemodynamic observations in evacuation of molar pregnancy. Am J Obstet Gynecol 138: 6–10, 1980.
5. Curry SL, Hammond CB, Tyrey L, Creasman WT, Parker RT: Hydatidiform mole: Diagnosis, management and long-term followup of 347 patients. Obstet Gynecol 45: 1–8, 1975.
6. French W, Freund U, Carlson RW, Weil MH: High output heart failure associated with pulmonary edema complicating hydatidiform mole. Arch Intern Med 137: 367–369, 1977.
7. Goldstein DP: Prophylactic chemotherapy of patients with molar pregnancy. Obstet Gynecol 38: 817–822, 1971.
8. Hendrickse JPD, Willis AJP, Evans KT: Acute dyspnoea with trophoblastic tumours. J Obstet Gynaecol Br Commw 72: 376–383, 1965.
9. Higgins HP, Hershman JM, Kenimer JG, Patillo RA, Bayley A, Walfish P: The thyrotoxicosis of hydatidiform mole. Ann Intern Med 83: 307–311, 1975.
10. Higgins HP, Herschmann JM: The hyperthyroidism due to trophoblastic hormone. Clin Endocrinol Metab 7: 307–311, 1978.
11. Huberman RP, Fon GT, Bein ME: Benign molar pregnancies: Pulmonary complications. Am J Roentgenol 138: 71–74, 1982.
12. Kohorn EI, McGinn RC, Gee JBL, Goldstein DP, Osathanondh R: Pulmonary embolization of trophoblastic tissue in molar pregnancy. Obstet Gynecol 51: 165–205, 1978.
13. Kohorn EI: Hydatidiform mole and gestational trophoblastic disease in southern Connecticut. Obstet Gynecol 59: 78–84, 1982.
14. Lipp RG, Kindschi JD, Schmitz R: Death from pulmonary embolism associated with hydatidiform mole. Am J Obstet Gynecol 83: 1644–1647, 1962.
15. Morrow CP, Kletzky OA, Disaia PJ, Townsend DE, Mishell DR, Nakamura RM: Clinical and laboratory correlates of molar pregnancy and trophoblastic disease. Am J Obstet Gynecol 128: 424–430, 1977.
16. Orr JW, Austin JM, Hatch KD, Shingleton HM, Younger JB, Boots LR: Acute pulmonary edema associated with molar pregnancies: A high risk factor for development of persistent trophoblastic disease. Am J Obstet Gynecol 136: 412–415, 1980.
17. Pritchard JA: Blood volume changes in pregnancy and the puerperium. Am J Obstet Gynecol 91: 621–627, 1965.
18. Romero R, Horgan JG, Kohorn EI, Kadar N, Taylor KJW, Hobbins JC: New criteria for the diagnosis of gestational trophoblastic disease. Obstet Gynecol (submitted for publication).
19. Trotter RF, Tieche HL: Maternal death due to pulmonary embolism of trophoblastic cells. Am J Obstet Gynecol 71: 1114–1118, 1956.
20. Twiggs LB, Morrow CP, Schlaerth JB: Acute pulmonary complications of molar pregnancy. Am J Obstet Gynecol 135: 189–194, 1979.
21. Twiggs LB: Nonneoplastic complications of molar pregnancy. Clin Obstet Gynecol 27: 199–210, 1984.

14

Hydatidiform Mole: Data from a Series of 5124 Cases in the United Kingdom

Joan Dent and K. D. Bagshawe

During the 1960s it bacame clear that despite the identification of hydatidiform mole (HM) patients as a high-risk group and despite major improvements in the treatment of invasive mole and choriocarcinoma, some patients still died from its sequelae. One reason for this was the difficulty of maintaining effective follow-up from busy clinical units, leading to delay in diagnosis of choriocarcinoma. Another problem was that the sequelae to HM present a great variety of features, yet most obstetricians saw only a limited number of patients with HM. Therefore it was difficult for individual obstetricians to know when and whether therapeutic intervention was required.

One approach has been to give cytotoxic chemotherapy, or so-called prophylactic chemotherapy, to all patients with HM. Another more selective approach has been to give chemotherapy to any patient whose serum or urine concentration of human chorionic gonadotropin (hCG) has not fallen to undetectable levels within 4 to 6 weeks. This results in treating some 20 to 30% of all HM patients with chemotherapy. A third, still more selective approach has been to allow a longer period for hCG values to fall before instituting chemotherapy.

A hydatidiform mole registration scheme was established in 1973 under the auspices of the Royal College of Obstetricians and Gynaecologists and the Department of Health and Social Security to provide data about hydatidiform mole in the United Kingdom and to provide effective follow-up arrangements for patients with respect to possible invasive and malignant sequelae. The scheme is voluntary and is based on three registration and follow-up centers (Dundee, Sheffield, and London) and two treatment centers (Sheffield and London). In the 11-year period up to the end of 1983, a total of 8,095 patients were registered at the three centers. The present report is a preliminary analysis and evaluation of part of the data on 5124 patients registered at the London (Charing Cross) center between January 1973 and December 1983. More detailed evaluation of the data in the context of the existing literature will be published elsewhere.

METHODS

Under the registration scheme, a patient who had undergone evacuation of a clinically or pathologically identified hydatidiform mole was reported to one of the registration/follow-up centers using a standard registration form. The decision as to whether a conception resulted in HM requiring follow-up rested with the referring gynecologist or pathologist. Histological slides or blocks were requested for examination at the Charing Cross Hospital for all patients who required chemotherapy and, since 1982, for all registered patients whether or not chemotherapy was required.

The registration form requested the name, date of birth, ethnic group, ABO and Rh blood groups of the patient and her partner, obstetric history, mode of evacuation of the HM, and history of the HM pregnancy and use of oral contraceptives prior to the HM. The classification of HM used in 1973 was 1) classical or complete HM (CHM); 2) transitional; and 3) molar degeneration. The designation transitional was later replaced by partial HM (PHM) to conform with current usage and advances in the cytogenetic definition of CHM and PHM. In 1983 a request was sent to the referring gynecologist asking permission to request additional information from the patient. When this permission was obtained, additional information relating to the obstetric history and the use of oral contraceptives or other forms of estrogen/progestogen therapy was requested because early experience showed that this information when supplied by the medical attendant was often incomplete or inaccurate.

On receipt of the registration form, the registration center sent a letter of instructions to the patient. Following this a returnable, postage prepaid box containing sample tube for urine and/or serum was sent, which was to be returned to the registration center laboratory for estimation of hCG concentration. Samples were normally requested every 2 weeks until hCG values had fallen to the normal or undetectable range; then monthly up to 1 year postevacuation; then every 3 months until 2 years postevacuation. An additional two specimens were requested after any pregnancy subsequent to HM. The 2-year follow-up period was not regarded as mandatory in all patients. In particular, patients who wished to proceed with another pregnancy as soon as possible were advised that their risk of malignant sequelae to HM were very small when their hCG results were known to have been normal for 6 months. The criteria used for therapeutic intervention have been described elsewhere. In summary, they were 1) persisting high levels of hCG ($>$20,000 IU/liter hCG in serum) more than 4 weeks postevacuation; 2) histological evidence of choriocarcinoma; 3) evidence of metastases in brain, liver, gastrointestinal tract, or metastases $>$2 cm on chest x-ray; 4) persisting uterine hemorrhage; 5) persistently rising hCG values; or 6) hCG persisting in body fluids at any level 4 to 6 months postevacuation. If a patient seemed likely to require chemotherapy by these criteria, admission to Charing Cross Hospital was offered via the referring obstetrician.

The hCG level was measured in duplicate by double antibody radioimmunoassay [4] using Kemtek 3300 automated assay machines on serum or urine [1]. The sensitivity of the methods improved during the 11-year period mainly as a result of improvements of antibody characteristics. The current assay detects 1 to 5 IU/liter of hCG using antisera directed at β-hCG, and cross-reactivity with luteinizing hormone is $<1\%$. Values <4

IU/liter on serum or <24 IU/liter on urine have been regarded as "normal." The assay results were sent to the gynecologist and general practitioner and were recorded manually in serial form until 1980, since which time they were recorded on computer file. Registration dates have lagged behind evacuation dates, and the evacuation dates for 73 patients preceded the start of the registration scheme.

Referring gynecologists were able to register a patient with any of the three registration/follow-up centers, but there was a general trend toward registration on a geographical basis. Patients in Northern Ireland were originally registered and followed up in Belfast, but later were registered at Charing Cross Hospital.

The numbers of registered live births in England and Wales were obtained from the publications of the Office of Population and Census. The opportunity to check the validity of the information provided on the registration forms and by direct postal questionnaire was limited to those patients referred to Charing Cross Hospital for treatment or who, because of residence in the London area, attended our clinic. The obstetric history recorded on the registration forms and that obtained by careful direct interview of the patients were compared. Statistical analyses were performed by chi square using Pearson's tables.

RESULTS

Number of Registered Patients by Year

The number of patients registered annually at Charing Cross tended to increase progressively during the 11-year period (Table 1), and ranged from 331 in 1975 to 676 in 1983. Using the defined criteria for therapeutic intervention, the number of patients requiring treatment varied from year to year, but no consistent trend was seen. The number treated ranged from 21 in 1974 to 53 in 1982; the percentage of patients with HM evacuated in any year who required chemotherapy ranged from 5.41% in 1973 to 9.92% in 1979, with an overall figure of 7.75% (Table 1). Of the 397 treated patients, 391 were treated at Charing Cross Hospital and 6 were treated at other hospitals mostly using protocols advised by Charing Cross.

The age of patients at the time of evacuation of HM is shown in Table 2, together with the number of patients requiring treatment and the number of registered live births for the corresponding year in England and Wales.

Ethnic Groups

The ethnic groups of patients with HM are shown in Table 3. Details of the geographical distribution of different ethnic groups in the United Kingdom are not available, nor are the number of live births classified on an ethnic basis.

Table 1. Number of hydatidiform mole patients registered at Charing Cross Hospital by year

	Pre-1973	1973	1974	1975	1976	1977	1978	1979	1980	1981	1982	1983	Total	Mean
Registered		363	335	331	388	460	422	485	482	542	640	676	5,124	466
Evacuated	73	355	328	350	384	442	435	494	482	542	629	610	5,124	466
Treated	4	34	21	33	28	29	37	49	40	36	53	33	397	36
Percent treated	5.5	9.58	6.4	9.43	7.29	6.56	8.50	9.92	8.3	6.64	8.43	5.41	7.75	
Live birth*		676	640	603	584	569	596	638	656	634	626	629	6,851	623

* Number of live births recorded in England and Wales in thousands for the corresponding years.

Table 2. Patients' age at time of evacuation of hydatidiform mole (yr), number and percent treated, annual number of live births in England and Wales by age, ratio of hydatidiform mole to live births by age, and relative risk

	<15	15–19	20–24	25–29	30–34	35–39	40–44	45–49	>50	Unknown
No. with HM	11	646	1,376	1,597	828	351	138	106	70	1 (unknown)
No. treated by chemotherapy	1	37	107	140	57	19	11	12	13	397 (total)
Percent	9.1	5.7	7.8	8.8	6.9	5.4	8.0	11.3	18.6	7.75 (mean)
Live births*	254	61,152	174,504	222,873	106,238	30,190	6,475	564	24	
No. of live births/no. of HM	23.1	94.7	126.8	139.6	128.3	86.0	46.9	5.3	0.34	
Relative risk per pregnancy compared with 25–29 yr age group†	6.04	1.47	1.10	1.00	1.09	1.62	2.97	26.3	411	

The mean number of live births per annum was obtained for the period 1973–1981 except for those <15 years and those >50 years (5- and 6-year data used, respectively).

* Mean number of live births in England and Wales per year, 1973 through 1983.

† Relative risk was calculated by dividing the number of live births in England and Wales by the corresponding number of HM in each group: the relative risk for each group was related to the 25–29 year age group, which was assigned a risk value of 1.0.

Table 3. Ethnic groups of patients with hydatidiform mole

Ethnic group*	No. of cases	No. of cases treated	Percent treated
European/Caucasian	4,190	355	8.5
Black	136	12	8.8
Asian (Indian, Chinese, Southeast Asian)	356	27	7.6
Not defined	472	3	0.06
Total	5,124	397	7.75

* Patients admitted for treatment were all classified into one of the first three categories except for three patients who were treated elsewhere.

Table 4. ABO blood group of patients with hydatidiform mole

Blood group	Total no. of cases	No. of cases treated	Percent treated*
A	2,013	158	7.85
O	2,119	180	8.49
AB	154	11	7.14
B	504	47	9.32
Unknown	334	1	0.30

* Differences between the percentage treated in the known blood groups is not significant.

Table 5. Classification of mole by histopathological examination at treatment center and no. requiring chemotherapy in a group of 317 patients registered for hydatidiform mole in 1983

	Total no. of cases	No. of cases treated	Percent treated
Complete HM	210	18	8.6
Partial HM	51	0	—
HM of uncertain type; suspected HM	54	3	5.7
Not HM	2		
Total	317	21	6.6

Blood Group Data

Patient ABO groups are shown in Table 4. The ABO groups of the patients' partners are not listed as the data available for the patients' partners was strongly influenced by the patient being referred for treatment.

Histopathology

Throughout the study, material for histopathological examination was requested for all cases requiring treatment. No analysis of this material is presented here. During 1982 we began to request material for histological examination on all registered patients. The analysis here is restricted to 317 patients for whom material was made available for histological examination during 1983. The material was reviewed at the registration center by one of us (KDB) and the classification compared with that of the pathologist at the referring hospital. There was agreement on histopathological classification in 191 instances, disagreement in 45, and some uncertainty in both opinions in 81. The analysis of the material at the referring center is shown in Table 5. Cases classified as probable CHM or probable PHM were classified as complete or partial, respectively.

Additional information from referring centers indicated that there were 24 cases of HM with fetus, which may have been twin pregnancies. Three of these patients required

Table 6. Pregnancies before first registered hydatidiform mole

	No.	Percent
No recorded prior pregnancy	1,950	(38)
One or more prior pregnancies	3,174	(62)
No previous live birth	2,406	(47)
One or more prior live births	2,717	(53)
One or more prior stillbirths	44	(0.86)
No recorded prior abortion	3,836	(75)
One or more prior abortions	1,264	(25)
Prior HM	21	(0.66)

* The stillbirth rate for England and Wales was 0.97% of live births in 1976, and fell progressively to 0.57% in 1983 (OPCS data).

Table 7. Mode of mole evacuation as defined by referring gynecologist

Mode of evacuation	Total no. of cases	No. of cases treated	Percent treated	p
Spontaneous+D & C	1,374	47	3.42	<0.001
Suction+D & C	1,443	122	8.45	
Medical induction+D & C	640	94	14.7	<0.005
Hysterectomy	62	5	8.06	
Hysterectomy+SO	23	0	—	
Hysterotomy	29	6	20.7	<0.05
Salpingectomy+D & C	37	0	—	
D & C only	1,461	122	8.35	
Not defined	55	1	1.82	
Total	5,124	397	7.75	

D & C=dilatation and curettage; medical induction=oxytocin or prostaglandin induction; SO=unilateral or bilateral salpingectomy and oophorectomy.

treatment. In addition, there were six cases of HM with live births, one of whom required treatment.

Obstetric History

Recorded obstetric histories from the registration forms are summarized in Table 6.

Mode of Evacuation

The methods of evacuation used in the series are summarized in Table 7, together with the number and percentage of patients in each category who required chemotherapy. There were 37 patients who were identified as having tubal moles removed by salpingectomy.

Human Chorionic Gonadotropin

Under the registration scheme, first samples of urine or serum were not taken until several days, or in some cases several weeks, after evacuation of the HM. At the time of evacuation, 203 patients had hCG values >100,000 IU/liter in serum or urine. Of these, 25 (12.3%) required treatment. On the day of evacuation, 98 patients had hCG values <100,100 IU/liter, and 6 (6.1%) of these required treatment. It is likely that there was a selective effect influencing these data so that they cannot be regarded as representative of the whole series.

The fall in hCG levels following evacuation of HM was analyzed for 4,205 patients. Patients treated for invasive mole or choriocarcinona, defaulters and late registrations were excluded. Normal hCG values were not attained until 20–22 weeks post-evacuation in 3% of patients and 0.3% of patients had abnomal values of hCG 30–32 weeks post-evacuation of HM but did not require chemotherpy (Figure 1).

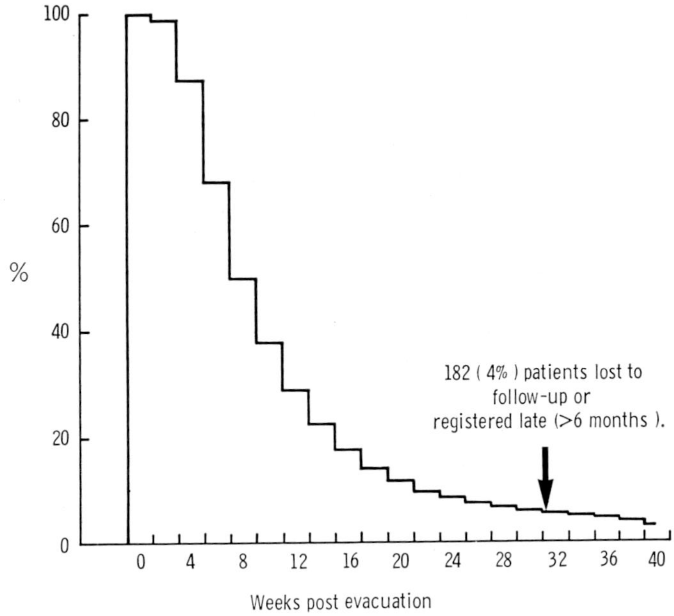

Figure 1. Time for hCG to reach normal concentration in 4,205 patients registered at the Charing Cross Hospital for follow-up after HM (1973–1983)

Table 8. Pregnancies subsequent to registered hydatidiform mole*

	No. of cases	Percent
One or more subsequent pregnancies	2,657	(52)
One or more subsequent live births	2,354	(46)
One or more subsequent aboritions	509	
Subsequent hydatidiform moles	47	
Subsequent stillbirths	21	(0.4)
Subsequent pregnancy, unknown outcome	45	(0.9)
Total no. of pregnancies recorded	3,692	

* Pregnancies subsequent to first registered hydatidiform mole through March 22, 1985.

Known pregnancies occurring subsequent to evacuation of HM are shown in Table 8.

Repeat Mole

Data relating to patients who had more than one HM are summarized and tabulated in Table 9. The data were revised up to March 23, 1985.

Oral Contraceptives

Retrospective analysis revealed that 151 patients reported using oral contraceptives within 6 months of evacuation of HM and while they were known to have elevated hCG concentrations in serum or urine. Of these patients, 68 (45%) required treatment by the criteria applied throughout the series. No breakdown of the form of oral contraception used by these patients has been attempted, but these figures include three patients given medroxyprogesterone (Depo-Provera) immediately after the evacuation of HM. All three of these patients required chemotherapy. An additional patient used oral contraceptives

Table 9. Repeat moles

	No. of patients	
a. History of HM anteceding first registered HM	21	
One HM subsequent to first registered HM	45	
Two HM subsequent to first registered HM	2	
One HM anteceding first registered HM and one HM subsequent to first registered HM	4	
Total no. with 2 HM	64	
Total no. with 3 HM	8	
Total no. with repeated moles	72	
Two consecutive HM pregnancies (among 72 patients)	45	
b. Patients with one or more pregnancy following first HM	2,657	
Total pregnancies recorded followed first HM	3,692	
Incidence of second HM per patient at risk		1 : 52
Incidence of second HM per pregnancy at risk		1 : 76
c. Patients with one or more pregnancies following second HM	38	
Patients with one or more live births following second HM	29	
No. of pregnancies in patients following second HM		
Outcome—Live births	52	
Abortions	36	
Third HM	6	
Unknown	2	
Incidence of third HM per patient at risk		1 : 4.75
Incidence of third HM per pregnancy at risk		1 : 6.5
d. Patients with pregnancies following third HM	2	
Outcome—Live births	1	
Abortions	1	

Five of the eight patients who had a third HM had no successful pregnancy.

Table 10. Causes of death

	No. of cases
Pulmonary embolism at reevacuation of HM	2
Accidental death (1 traffic accident; 1 overdose)	2
Intraabdominal hemorrhage 3 months postevacuation (patient abroad)	1
Cerebrovascular hemorrhage after subsequent live birth	1
Intercurrent lymphoma	1
Acute hepatic failure 2 weeks after completing chemotherapy for metastatic disease, hepatitis B+ve	1
Myocardial infarction during chemotherapy	1
Drug resistance	2

after HM and her 3-month-postevacuation hCG estimation proved normal. She subsequently delivered a second HM and then required treatment.

Another 548 patients used oral contraceptives or medroxyprogesterone within 6 months of evacuation of HM after hCG concentrations in serum or urine had reached normal values. Three of these patients (0.55%) required treatment. One of these patients was treated 32 months after evacuation of HM and after two intervening abortions. One was treated 31 months postevacuation of HM after an intervening live birth. The third was treated for rising hCG values 18 months after HM. There were 527 patients reporting that they had never used oral contraceptives, and 58 of these (11.01%) required treatment.

Deaths

There were 11 deaths (0.2%) among the 5,124 registered patients. The causes of death are summarized in Table 10.

DISCUSSION

The United Kingdom registration scheme has been well supported by obstetricians. However, we have no reliable guide to the completeness of ascertainment of the scheme.

The progressive increase in the numbers of patients with HM registered annually (Table 1) could reflect an increasing incidence of HM or a greater use of the registration scheme. As there has been no corresponding change in the number of patients requiring treatment despite the use of standardized criteria for treatment, it seems possible that the criteria for identifying aborted conceptuses as HM has changed during the 11-year period. Major factors contributing to this may be a greater tendency to err on the side of caution and the relative convenience of the follow-up service and availability of hCG assays. However, the possibility of increased incidence of CHM, PHM, or both cannot be excluded by the present analysis.

The percentage of patients treated each year has varied between 5.41% and 9.92%. In addition to difficulties in identifying HM, there may have been some variation in rigorousness with which the criteria used to select patients for treatment were applied. Although the indications defined in the introduction have been adhered to, an element of clinical judgment enters with patients who have elevated hCG values 4 to 6 months postevacuation. Different members of the clinical team may have applied different thresholds.

Clearly the possibility of identifying patients who do not need follow-up after HM merits careful study and it will be important to establish the level of risk, if any, of choriocarcinoma after PHM.

The data provide a broad guide to the incidence of HM in the United Kingdom.

In drawing conclusions from this, due regard must be paid to the limitations of the data, particularly in classifying borderline cases as HM and the uncertainty regarding the incorporation of all HMs in the United Kingdom into the registration scheme. Also, the total number of aborted pregnancies is unknown and histological examination of products of conception was not consistently performed.

The mean number of registered cases in England and Wales for the 11-year period 1973 through 1983 was 622 per year, with a range of 502 to 970 a year. These figures were derived by excluding registrations at the Dundee, Scotland, center and in Northern Ireland from the total number of registrations. The mean number of live births in England and Wales for the same period was 623,000 per annum. On this basis the incidence of registered HMs was 0.998 per 1,000 live births. In 1983 the number of registered HMs totaled 970 and live births totaled 636,000, giving an incidence of 1.525 per 1,000 live births. In so far as the registration scheme is incomplete, the ratio of moles to live births would be higher. Because of the difficulties of identifying some HMs, the registration is incomplete and that of PHMs is probably more incomplete than that for CHMs. On the basis of the histological evidence from a sample (317) of the cases registered in 1983 (Table 5), the ratio of CHMs to live births in England and Wales was 1:973. Exclusion of nonmoles from the registration data would conversely tend to lower the ratio, but the number and effect of these is small.

These figures suggest that HM is more prevalent than had been previously suspected. The evidence may support a suspicion that the incidence is increasing. Other data sources for the incidence of HM in the United Kingdom are few, but a recent study in one region gave an incidence of 0.65 HM per 1,000 deliveries [3]. On the other hand, the absence of a corresponding trend in the number of patients requiring chemotherapy may reflect differences arising in the criteria for registration or may reflect improvement in methods of primary management. An earlier analysis [4, 5] suggested that the mode of evacuation of HM and estrogens or progestogens taken postevacuation while hCG was still detectable in serum or urine may have modified clinical practice.

The age of patients with HM (Table 2) shows the expected increased risk for pregnancies in older age groups, but these data reveal the magnitude of this excess. There is a progressive increase in risk with increasing age so that for women aged over 50 years the risk of a pregnancy resulting in mole was 411 times greater than the risk of HM in women aged 25 to 29 years. Evidence of increased risk of HM in younger age groups has been suspected from previous studies, but the data here reveal only a slight excess risk in the 15 to 19 year age group, where the risks are comparable to those aged 35 to 39 years. However, pregnancies occurring in patients under 15 years old carried a six-fold increase in risk compared with those in patients aged 25 to 29 years.

The ethnic groups of patients indicate that 18.8% of registered patients were non-Caucasian. As there are no data recording live births by ethnic group in the United Kingdom, we cannot determine whether there is racial predisposition to HM within the population subgroups resident in the United Kingdom. These patients whose ethnic group was not defined included a high proportion of patients of Chinese, Southeast Asian, and mixed racial origin. Data from the Office of Population Censuses and Surveys indicated that for the years 1973 through 1983 between 11.5% and 13.2% of all live births in England and Wales were to women born outside the United Kingdom.

A previous analysis of blood group data from the Charing Cross series showed marked effects in patients treated for trophoblastic tumors, particularly where these followed live births or nonmole abortions. No marked trends were seen in relation to patients with HM. The present data tend to confirm this conclusion, but a more detailed analysis will be presented elsewhere.

It is also significant that during the period of data collection, 1973 through 1983, the genetic and morphological criteria for distinguishing CHM and PHM have been clarified. Nevertheless, not all histopathologists are fully aware of the developments in this area, and it can be argued that the criteria for diagnosing HM are still too arbitrary to permit a confident diagnosis in all suspected cases. The borderlands of hydropic change and HM are difficult to define.

Since 1983 an attempt has been made to independently review the histological material for all registered cases. Material for histological examination was made available for 317 of 676 cases in 1983. Although in the majority of cases (60.2%) both the local pathologist and one of the authors (KDB) agreed as to the histological diagnosis, there was no agreement in 14.2% of cases and doubt about the lesion in 25.6% of cases.

Overall, 7.75% of all registered cases were treated with chemotherapy. After complete HM in the histologically reviewed 1983 series, 7.9% were treated; after PHM in the reviewed 1983 series there were no patients requiring treatment. However, individual patients who have had PHM have been treated for trophoblastic lesions, and in at least one case there was evidence consistent with metastatic choriocarcinoma. It is not established whether this arose from the PHM or another pregnancy.

As the risk of requiring chemotherapy for invasive mole or postmole choriocarcinoma is much greater after CHM than after PHM, and somewhat greater than after HM of undefined type, the proportion of the different categories of HM in a series has a marked influence on the proportion requiring chemotherapy. Similarly the criteria for intervention with chemotherapy have a marked effect. In general the policy adopted in the United Kingdom and elsewhere in Europe has been not to intervene as long as there is a high probability that the HM will die spontaneously. In North America and elsewhere therapeutic intervention has been the rule when hCG has persisted in body fluids for 4 to 6 weeks, and in some cases intervention occurs earlier on the basis of prognostic criteria. In contrast with other series where 20% to 30% of HM patients receive chemotherapy, less than 8% of patients in this series required chemotherapy. This suggests that in North America it is common practice to give cytotoxic agents to patients with lesions that would otherwise resolve spontaneously or that clinical practices favor a higher rate of malignant or potentially malignant sequelae.

The obstetric history of patients as recorded on the registration forms proved to have a poor level of accuracy when compared with the history obtained by personal interview. Personal interview was largely restricted to patients in the London area and to all patients who were referred for chemotherapy. Even with this limitation, certain conclusions can be drawn. Almost half the patients (47%) had no live term birth prior to the HM and 25% had a prior abortion.

A previous analysis suggested that the method of evacuation of HM could have a marked effect on the subsequent need for chemotherapy [5, 6]. Methods that resulted in handling or contraction of the uterus appeared less favorable. Since that report medical induction and hysterotomy have been less used in the United Kingdom than formerly, but the present data support the previous evidence that medical induction and hysterotomy are more likely to have sequelae requiring chemotherapy than other methods. Alternatively it can be argued that the pathological state requiring the use of medical induction or hysterotomy are the factors responsible for these differences.

There were 72 patients in the series who had more than one HM. Eight of these had three HMs, and the remainder had two HMs. There were 21 patients that had a HM before their first registered HM, and 45 that had a HM afterwards. Data on the risk of a second HM pregnancy have not been available or have been based on comparatively small series. The risk of a pregnancy after HM resulting in a second HM in this series was 1: 76. The risk of a third HM in patients at risk was 1: 6.5.

Thus, although the risk of a second mole is probably 10- to 20-fold higher than that of a first HM, the majority of patients who wanted an additional pregnancy had a successful live birth. Obviously this number will continue to increase throughout the child-bearing period of the registered cases. Even in patients that had two HMs the chances of a subsequent live birth are good, as 29 of 38 (76%) such patients were successful. For patients who have had three HMs the data are too few to draw conclusions. However, it is noted that one of two subsequent pregnancies resulted in a live birth, although five of eight patients who had three HMs had no successful pregnancy.

The interval between evacuation of HM and the date when hCG was known to be normal or undetectable in patients who did not require chemotherapy showed a distribution similar to that previously observed in this and other series. It is notable that in a few patients hCG did not reach undetectable levels until 24 to 32 weeks postevacuation. These patients did not appear to be more prone to relapse than those attaining normal values earlier, but the number of such patients is small.

The 11 deaths recorded in the series resulted from eight different causes. Two patients died of progressive choriocarcinoma that became drug resistant. Two died from complications of hydatidiform mole. One of these was the wife of a British soldier in Europe, and the first sample to reach the laboratory indicated a high concentration of hCG 8 weeks postevacuation, which we regard as a warning of possible uterine perforation from invasive mole or choriocarcinoma. Death might have been avoided if samples had been received earlier.

The scheme has not been able to prevent all deaths attributable to sequelae to HM. However, the fatality rate of 0.2% from all causes was attributed to unrelated causes in 4 cases and was probably due to unrelated causes in 5 of 11 cases, so the fatality rate attributable to HM was close to 0.1%.

The estimated cost of the scheme has been analyzed in an earlier report [2] in relation to the estimated cost benefits resulting from avoidance of treating patients with advanced disease. On this basis it was concluded that it is less expensive than not to run such a scheme in terms of total health care.

SUMMARY

Between 1973 and 1983 a total of 5,124 patients were registered at Charing Cross Hospital, London, for HM. This paper presented a preliminary analysis of some of the data.

The incidence of HM in England and Wales for the 11-year period from 1973 through 1983 was close to 1 per 1,000 live births. The number of cases registered tended to increase, and for 1983 the incidence of HM was 1.525 per 1,000 live births. The incidence of CHM in the United Kingdom in 1983 was estimated to be 1.027 per 1,000 live births. In a sample of 317 patients registered in 1983, 16.0% were classified as having PHM and 66% as having CHM.

The incidence of HM in relation to live births was markedly age dependent, being lowest at 25 to 29 years. The risk per pregnancy increased with age and over 50 years, and was 411 times greater than for the 25 to 29 year age group. Pregnency under the age of 15 years carried a six times greater risk of HM than that for the 25 to 29 year age group.

Overall, 7.75% of the registered patients were treated with chemotherapy for invasive mole or choriocarcinoma. The remainder regressed without chemotherapy. Patients who had medical induction with oxytocin or prostaglandins or who underwent hysterotomy had a higher risk of requiring chemotherapy subsequently.

There were no live births before HM was evacuated in 47% of the patients registered, and 25% reported a prior spontaneous or surgical abortion. In 46% of the patients there were one or more live birth following HM.

Chemotherapy was not required by 3.2% of patients who still had elevated hCG values 20 to 22 weeks after evacuation of HM.

The risk of a pregnancy after a first HM resulting in a second HM was 1 : 76. One in 52 patients had a second HM. Of 38 patients who had additional pregnancies after a second HM, 29 had one or more subsequent live births, but eight had a third HM. The risk of a pregnancy resulting in a third HM after two HM pregnancies was 1 : 6.5. The incidence of third HM per patient at risk was 1 : 4.5. Of eight patients who had three HMs, five had no successful pregnancy.

Oral contraceptive use, or taking some form of estrogen/progestogen, during the 6-month period following evacuation of HM was reported by 699 patients. In 548 of these patients hCG levels had fallen to normal before steroid therapy was started, and three of these patients (0.55%) subsequently required chemotherapy. Of 151 patients taking steroids while hCG levels were still elevated, 68 (45%) required chemotherapy.

There were 11 deaths in the series (0.2%). Two of these deaths were from drug resistance.

ACKNOWLEDGMENTS

These studies were supported by the Cancer Research Campaign and the Medical Research Council.

REFERENCES

1. Bagshawe KD: Computer controlled automated radioimmunoassay. Lab Practice September 1975.
2. Bagshawe KD: Choriocarcinoma. Can we afford to cure cancer? Ann R Coll Surg Engl 60: 36–41, 1978.
3. Elston CW: The epidemiology of hydatidiform mole in Nottingham. Abstracts of International Symposium on Gestational Trophoblastic Tumours, London, 1976.
4. Kardana A, Bagshawe KD: A rapid, sensitive and specific radioimmunoassay for human chorionic gonadotrophin. J Immunol Methods 9: 297, 1976.
5. Stone M, Dent J, Kardana A, Bagshawe KD: Relationship of oral contraception to development of trophoblastic tumour after evacuation of a hydatidiform mole. Br J Obstet Gynaecol 83: 913–916, 1976.
6. Stone M, Bagshawe KD: An analysis of the influences of maternal age, gestational age, contraceptive method and the primary mode of treatment of patients with hydatidiform moles on the incidence of subsequent chemotherapy. Br J Obstet Gynaecol 86: 782–792, 1979.

15

Indications for Chemotherapy after Evacuation of Hydatidiform Mole: Length of Plateau of hCG Level Necessary for Diagnosis of Nonmetastatic Trophoblastic Neoplasia

Ernest I. Kohorn

At a time when no effective therapy beyond hysterectomy was available for gestational trophoblastic disease, classification was based on morphologic criteria. Now that effective chemotherapy is available even for advanced neoplasia, the disease is divided into groups that help indicate managements [1, 5, 6]. This clinical classification indicates the vigor with which therapy needs to be given. The level of human chorionic gonadotropin (hCG) correlates accurately with tumor load and provides the main indicator for monitoring therapy. Histology has thus become a secondary factor. The disease entities previously classified as invasive mole or chorioadenoma destruens may now be treated as nonmetastatic trophoblastic neoplasia without necessarily obtaining histologic confirmation of that diagnosis [7].

It is of note that the frequency of therapy in posthydatidiform mole patients (Table 1) appears to be higher than the incidence of choriocarcinoma and other malignant sequelae of hydatidiform mole in the prechemotherapy era (Table 2) [3]. This early administration of chemotherapy seems at variance with the known experience that chemotherapy for nonmetastatic neoplasia commenced within 16 weeks of mole evacuation is associated with a high cure rate in patients with hCG values of less than 50,000 mIU/mL of hCG-β.

The studies of Currie et al. [2] and Morrow et al. [10] have demonstrated a higher risk for trophoblastic sequelae if the uterus is enlarged by more than 4 weeks of gestational age or if theca-lutein cysts are present, and particularly if both factors are present together. Data from the Yale Center [9] and from Dallas Texas [14] show an increased association of each of these factors separately, but no greater increased risk for neoplasia with both these factors (Table 3) [9]. The incidence of uterine bleeding following mole evacuation is also higher among patients who require chemotherapy [2, 10], but bleeding after mole

Table 1. Trophoblastic sequelae after hydatidiform mole: Chemotherapy for persistently elevated hCG levels

	No. of cases	Sequelae	Percent	Center [Ref.]
	337	69	20	Duke [2]
	121	32	26	USC [10]
	212	68	32	Alabama
	100	15	15*	Boston [5]
	50	7	14†	Dallas [14]
	128	34	26	Yale [9]
Total	948	225	23.7	

* Selected group not treated with prophylactic chemotherapy.
† Only cases diagnosed by sonar.

Table 2. Trophoblastic sequelae in prechemotherapy era*

Total no. of patients with hydatidiform mole	129
Patients undergoing primary hysterectomy	10
Patients reaching undetectable levels of hCG	108
Patients with persistently elevated titers; hysterectomy performed—two died of choriocarcinoma	11
Incidence of trophoblastic neoplasia	21/129 (16%)

* Data from Delfs: Ann NY Acad Sci 80: 125, 1959

Table 3. Relation of uterine size, presence of theca-lutein cysts, and chemotherapy treatment after evacuation of hydatidiform mole

Center [Ref.]	No. of cases	Sequelae (%)*	With cyst (%)†	With enlarged uterus (%)†	Both (%)†
Yale [9]	128	34 (26)	12 (35)	16 (53)‡	7 (23)
Duke [2]	347	69 (20)	23 (49)‡	38 (55)‡	19 (57)
USC [10]	121	32 (26)	18 (56)	22 (69)	16 (50)
Dallas [14]	50	7 (14)	3 (35)	5 (71)	—

* Percent shown is of total no. of cases.
† Percent shown is of cases with sequelae.
‡ Cysts or an enlarged uterus were not evaluable in all cases.

evacuation may be a sign of incomplete evacuation and not necessarily an indicator of neoplasia.

Giving chemotherapy to the group of patients with such risk factors is only one step away from routine use of prophylactic chemotherapy. Prophylactic chemotherapy has been shown to reduce trophoblastic sequelae significantly [4], and metastatic sequelae particularly were much reduced. However, eight of ten patients would be treated unnecessarily. Kim et al. [8] have recently shown that prophylactic chemotherapy given to such a high-risk group of postmole patients may not prevent neoplasia, and elevated hCG levels requiring further chemotherapy may in fact present late. This implies that follow-up both by clinical observation and by hCG level monitoring is necessary even if prophylactic chemotherapy is given.

As hCG-β is a sensitive and accurate indicator of tumor load in trophoblastic disease [12], it would seem that this measure should be used as the sole indicator for initiating chemotherapy in asymptomatic patients who clearly do not have metastases and who may be followed up closely from week to week after mole evacuation. Among patient populations in whom close follow-up is not possible for social or logistic reasons, chemotherapy may be given for relative indications, assessed by the criteria of uterine size, bleeding of theca-lutein cysts, or embolization of molar tissue [11].

The selection of patients for chemotherapy after mole evacuation has been significantly

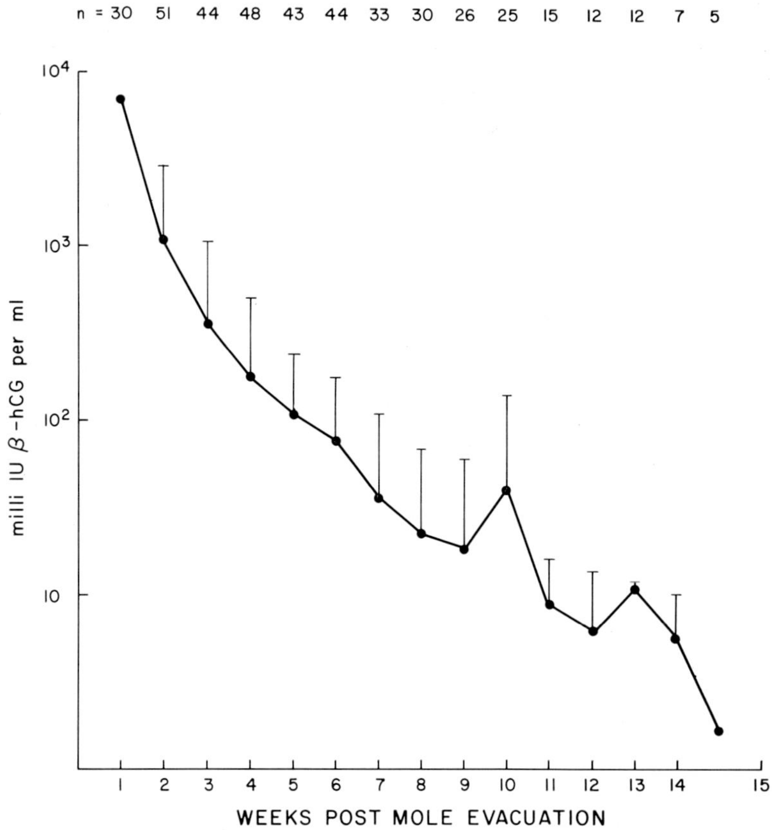

Figure 1. Regression of hCG-β after evacuation of hydatidiform mole in patients with no sequelae.

aided by reference to a curve of hCG values taken from patients with spontaneous regression of hCG after molar pregnancy (Figure 1) [9]. The use of such a graph was first suggested by Morrow et al. [10], who found that the values of hCG among patients who required chemotherapy were usually divergent from the "normal" regression curve by 4 weeks after mole evacuation. We have found a much greater variation in hCG regression after mole evacuation [9], and on occasion we could not discriminate abnormal values before 7 weeks postevacuation. By that time, however, high values rarely fell to nondetectable levels spontaneously. This time interval is still well within the "early" period for successful therapy of 16 weeks or less, as described by Ross et al. [13].

At present it is usual to make a diagnosis of nonmetastatic trophoblastic neoplasia after a plateau of three values of hCG over 2 weeks of observation. Chemotherapy is then initiated. Two weeks seems a short time of observation so early after mole evacuation, and it may be insufficiently long to justify a diagnosis of trophoblastic neoplasia and the administration of chemotherapy, particularly at levels of hCG-β of less than 1,000 mIU/mL.

Figure 2 shows an example of a patient in whom the hCG-β levels plateaued above 1,000 mIU/mL of hCG-β, and Figure 3 shows the values of two other patients with plateaus at levels above 100 mIU/mL. Both plateaus were transient, and in both patients hCG levels then declined spontaneously without therapy. Such plateaus are not infrequent and occurred 15 times among 195 patients seen with hydatidiform mole at Yale between 1971 and 1984 (Table 4).

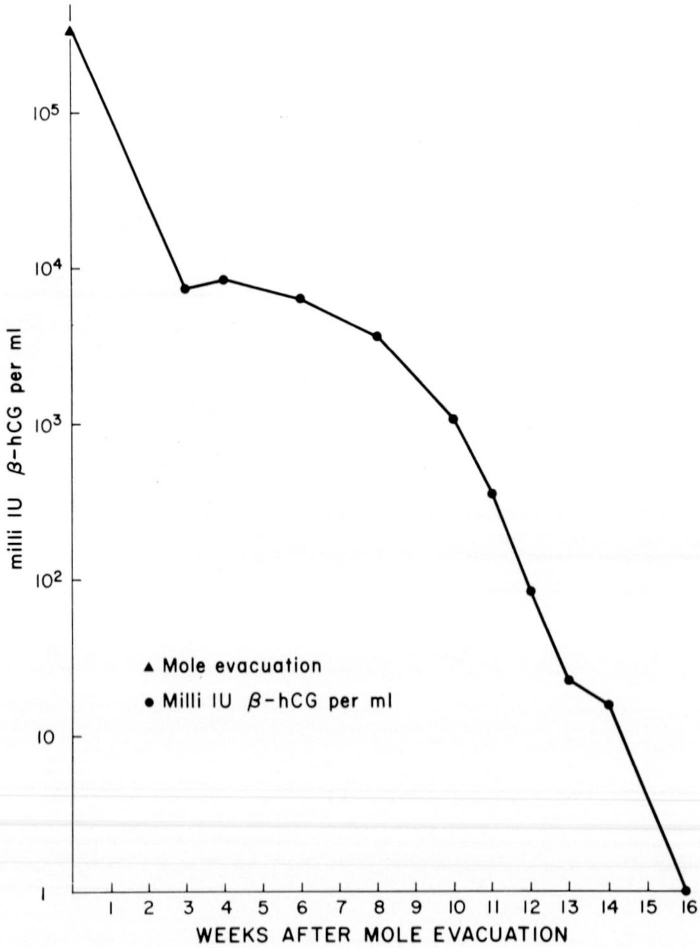

Figure 2. A plateau hCG-β level at greater than 10^3 mIU/mL at 3 weeks lasting 14 days, with subsequent uneventful fall without therapy.

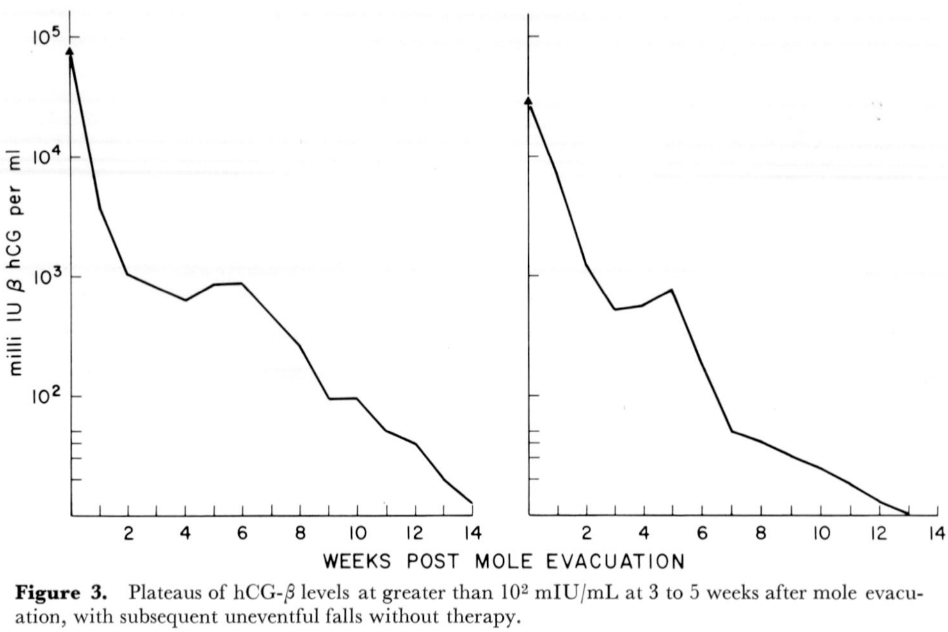

Figure 3. Plateaus of hCG-β levels at greater than 10^2 mIU/mL at 3 to 5 weeks after mole evacuation, with subsequent uneventful falls without therapy.

Table 4. Clinical diagnosis of patients seen at the Yale Center for Gestational Trophoblastic Disease (1971–1984)

Diagnosis		No.
Hydatidiform mole		195
Moles, no sequelae	124	
Moles, prophylactic chemotherapy	11	
Moles, with nonmetastatic trophoblastic neoplasia	53	
Moles, with metastatic trophoblastic neoplasia	7	
Choriocarcinoma uterus		5
Partial mole		16
Focus abnormal trophoblast in placenta		1
Ovarian hydatidiform mole		1
Total		218

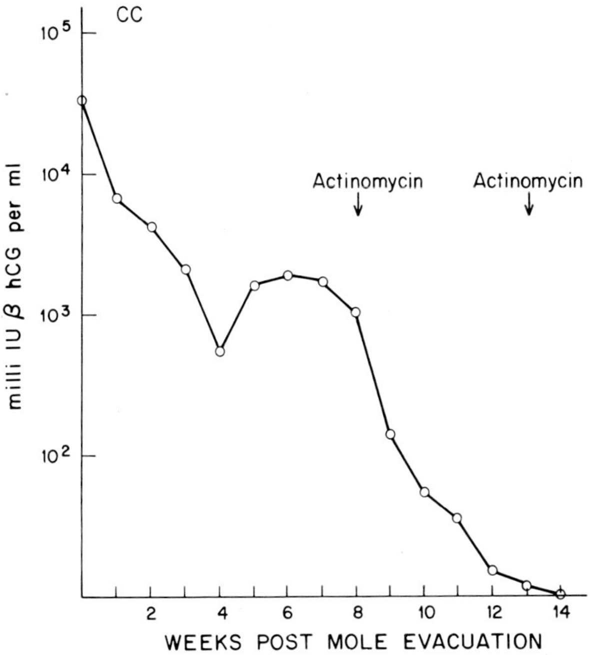

Figure 4. A plateau of hCG level 5 weeks after mole evacuation; four values over 4 weeks. Chemotherapy was commenced with subsequent remission.

It is suggested that in patients with values of hCG below 10^4 mIU/mL, hCG levels may be observed over 3 weeks (day x, x+7, x+14, x+21) before commencing chemotherapy, provided no other indicators for therapy such as metastases are present. Such practice should not prejudice the successful management of postmolar patients. By allowing a plateau to be present for 3 weeks within the first 12 weeks after mole evacuation, the clear need for therapy will have been demonstrated. By then there is likely to be little chance of spontaneous regression, but there is still an excellent chance for cure (Figure 4). With a plateau of hCG level of less than 10^3 mIU/mL, even 4 weeks may be allowed to elapse.

By implementing such a practice, the frequency of the diagnosis of nonmetastatic gestational trophoblastic disease will not be inflated because of a brief plateau of hCG-β level. This would provide a compromise between "neoprophylaxis" and ultraconservatism, and merits application in a larger group of patients.

ACKNOWLEDGMENT

This work was supported by the Baumer Fund of Yale University.

REFERENCES

1. Bagshawe KD: Risk and prognostic factors in trophoblastic neoplasia. Cancer 38: 1373–1385, 1976.
2. Currie SL, Hammond CB, Tyrey L, Creasman WT, Parker RT: Hydatidiform mole: Diagnosis, management and longterm follow up of 347 patients. Obstet Gynecol 45: 1–8, 1975.
3. Delfs E: Quantitative chorionic gonadotrophin: Prognostic value in hydatidiform mole and chorioepithelioma. Obstet Gynecol 9: 1–24, 1957.
4. Goldstein DP: The management of gestational trophoblastic disease. In Sturgis, Taylor (eds): Progress in Gynecology, vol. V. Grune & Stratton, New York, 1970.
5. Goldstein DP, Berkowitz RS: Management of gestational trophoblastic neoplasms. Curr Probl Obstet Gynecol 3: 1–47, 1980.
6. Hammond CB, Borchert LG, Tyrey L, Creasman WT, Parker RT: Treatment of metastatic trophoblastic disease: Good and poor prognosis. Am J Obstet Gynecol 115: 451–457, 1973.
7. Hatch KD, Shingleton HM, Austin JM, Boots LB, Younger JB, Soong SJ: Southern Regional Trophoblastic Disease Center, 1972–1977. South Med J 71: 1334–1336, 1978.
8. Kim KT, Hwang YY, Moon H, Kim DS: Effects of prophylactic chemotherapy on treatment and prognosis of hydatidiform mole. Proceedings of the Second World Congress on Trophoblastic Neoplasms, Singapore, 1984, p. 24.
9. Kohorn EI: Hydatidiform mole and gestational trophoblastic disease in Southern Connecticut: The experience of the Yale Center for Trophoblastic Disease. Obstet Gynecol 59: 78–84, 1982.
10. Morrow CP, Kletzky OA, DiSaia PJ, Townsend DE, Mishell DR, Nakamura RM: Clinical and laboratory correlates of molar pregnancy and trophoblastic disease. Am J Obstet Gynecol 128: 424–429, 1977.
11. Orr JW, Austin JM, Hatch KD, Shingleton HM, Younger JB, Boots LR: Acute pulmonary edema associated with molar pregnancy: A high-risk factor for development of persistent trophoblastic disease. Am J Obstet Gynecol 136: 412–415, 1980.
12. Patillo RA, Hussa RO, Ruckert ACF, Kurtz JW, Cade JM, Rinke ML: Human chorionic gonadotrophin in Be Wo trophoblastic cells after twelve years in continuous culture. Retention of intact human chorionic gonadotrophin secretion. Endocrinology 105: 967–974, 1979.
13. Ross GT, Goldstein DP, Hertz R, Lipsett MB, Odell WD: Sequential use of methotrexate and actinomycin D in the treatment of metastatic choriocarcinoma and related trophoblastic diseases in women. Am J Obstet Gynecol 93: 223–229, 1965.
14. Santos-Ramos R, Forney JP, Schwartz BE: Sonographic findings and clinical correlations in molar pregnancy. Obstet Gynecol 56: 186–192, 1980.

16

Histogenesis of Invasive Mole

Tsutomu Fukuschima

INTRODUCTION

The trophoblastic diseases involving hydatidiform moles, invasive moles, and choriocarcinomas are clinically treated as trophoblastic tumors, trophoblastic neoplasia, or chorionic lesions. In general, because hydatidiform mole, invasive mole, and choriocarcinoma seem to be considered as serial lesions according to clinical features, hydatidiform mole may be considered a neoplasia for convenience. On the other hand, some authors consider hydatidiform mole a trophoblastic hyperplasia, not a neoplasm [1]. Confusion may arise from a primary difference in viewpoint between the clinician and pathologist; therefore it is difficult to rely on experimental research to demonstrate choriocarcinoma from hydatidiform mole.

A conclusive view of these diseases still remains uncertain. However, clinically it is very important for therapy, follow-up, and prophylaxis whether or not to consider these diseases carcinogenic. As to the nature of hydatidiform mole, it is important to ascertain if it belongs to neoplasia, primary trophoblastic anomaly, or degeneration resulting from failed abortion. As to the origin of destructive mole, it is important to know whether it is an independent disease or a mutually dependent disease derived from hydatidiform mole.

Previous chromosomal studies by the author and coworkers have demonstrated that hydatidiform mole, invasive mole, and choriocarcinoma are not of independent origin, but are mutually dependent successive stages of malignant transformation. Also demonstrated was that the degree of chromosomal aberration tends to increase with increasing malignancy [3].

The present study examined whether there is a serial change from hydatidiform mole and from invasive mole to choriocarcinoma, and confirmed the above chromosomal findings about the relationship between hydatidiform mole and invasive mole.

MATERIAL AND METHODS

The study was carried out in 57 cases of invasive mole and more than 500 cases of hydatidiform mole, which were treated in the author's clinic during the past 15 years.

Observed uterus and tissues of invasive mole and hydatidiform mole were obtained by means of evacuation and hysterectomy. According to the diagnostic criteria used for classifying the differences of histogenesis, the hydatidiform moles were all typical moles, and did not include transitional moles or cystic degeneration of the placenta.

The invasive mole was myometrial invasion or growth in which villous structures were still identifiable in most specimens, which were collected before therapy. For the purpose of studying the relationship between mole tissue and its myometrium by histoanatomical observation, 30 uteri of hydatidiform mole obtained by hysterectomy without evacuation were rapidly fixed with 10% formalin and examined by histoanatomical study 1 week later. Three invasive moles were injected with opaque medium (Softex) through the uterine artery, then fixed by 10% formalin. Large sagittal sections were made 1 week later, and the macro-microhistological and vascular construction was studied by means of macroangiography.

RESULTS

We classified the grade of destructive features of the myometrium macrohistologically as follows: grade I—syncytial endometritis; grade II—elevated tumor formation in the uterine cavity; grade III—tumor formation within the uterine wall (including vascular embolized form); and grade IV—perforation (Table 1). There were 63 destructive features found in 57 cases; as noted in Table 1, three cases showed combined features of both grade III and grade IV. One of these cases with combined features is shown in Figure 3. As shown in the models in Figure 1, 40 features of grades II, III, and IV revealed definite destruction of the myometrium. On the other hand, 23 uteri showed only syncytial endometritis and were not remarkably destructive, although they had been diagnosed as invasive mole according to clinical evidence.

Grade II (elevated tumor formation in the uterine cavity) was considered the most

Table 1. Macrohistologic grading of destructive features of invasive mole

Grade and definition	No. of destructive features
I. Syncytial endometritis not remarkable for destruction	23
II. Elevated tumor formation in uterine cavity	22
III. Tumor formation within uterine wall* (including vascular embolized form)	13
VI. Perforation	5
Total	63

* Three cases showed combined features of both grade III and grade IV.

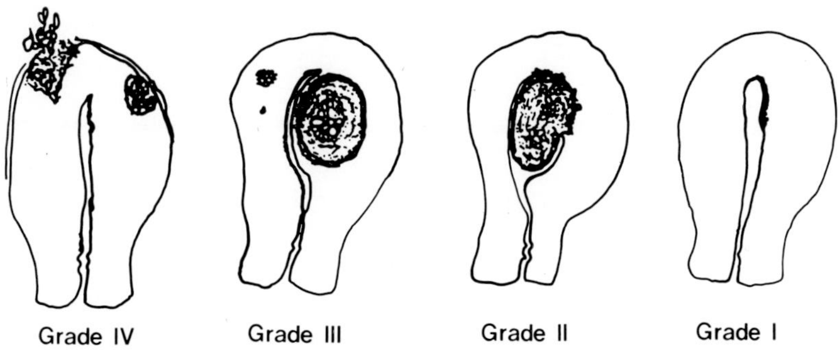

Figure 1. Models of macroscopical findings related to grades of destruction by destructive mole.

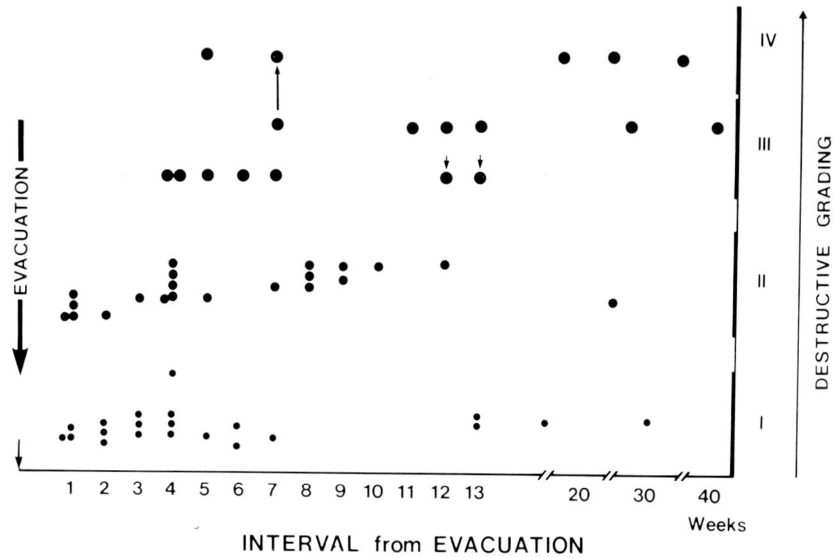

Figure 2. The relationship of grades of destruction by destructive mole based on macrohistological classification and the interval from evacuation of hydatidiform mole to hysterectomy of destructive mole.

frequent type, and was defined as 22 of 40 possible destructive features of the myometrium.

All cases of invasive moles studied occurred to some extent over a variable period of time after the evacuation of hydatidiform mole, which was the antecedent pregnancy. The longer the interval from evacuation to hysterectomy of the invasive mole, the higher the degree of destructive change in the myometrium (Figure 2). Histoanatomical observation revealed that 30 uteri containing hydatidiform mole tissue obtained by hysterectomy had various grades of destructive foci, or "radix" (Figure 4). These corresponded to the implantation site of the ovum.

COMMENTS

Based on many clinical reports and statistical studies on trophoblastic diseases, there is no doubt that hydatidiform mole bears a special relationship to invasive mole and chorio-

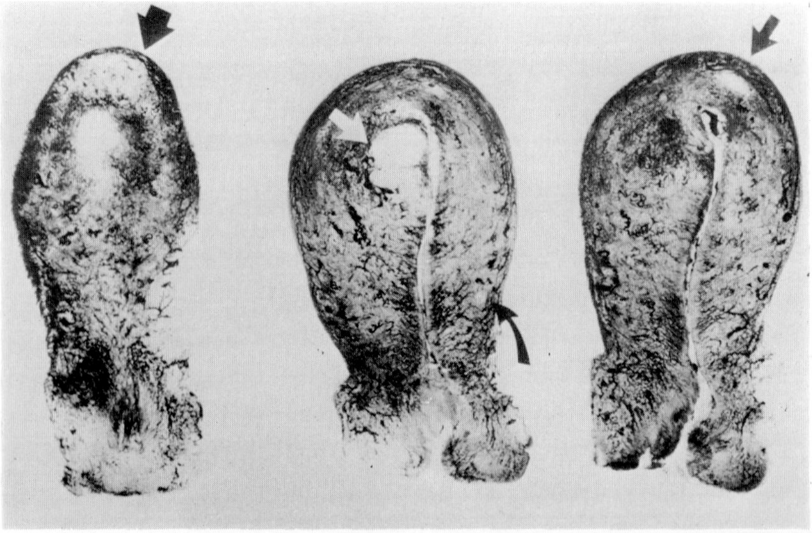

Figure 3. Combined features of both grade III and IV in destructive moles.

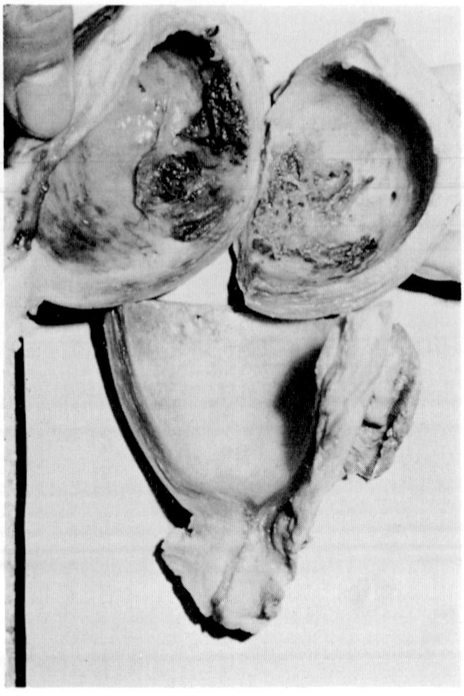

Figure 4. Various grades of destructive foci shown in hysterectomized uteri with hydatidiform mole.

carcinoma. Practically, it is convenient to treat these diseases, even hydatidiform mole, as trophoblastic neoplasia and spectrum diseases in the clinical field. The fact that the frequency of choriocarcinoma is decreased by the prophylactic use of methotrexate or preventive hysterectomy in mole patients may be supported by the consideration that choriocarcinoma is considered to arise from hydatidiform mole. However, to the contrary, some pathologists have emphasized the view that hydatidiform mole and destructive mole do not seem to warrant classification as neoplasms because they result from degeneration of chorionic villi and missed abortion of a blighted ovum. Considering them as spectrum diseases, the risk of choriocarcinoma following hydatidiform mole would be much more expected as a real probability. It is difficult to decide whether hydatidiform mole should most properly be regarded a result of degeneration, hyperplasia, dysplasia, or benign neoplasia of the trophoblast. Thus the line of demarcation in the clinical sense is now so blurred as to consider hydatidiform mole as neoplasia.

On the other hand, studies on the histological characteristics and growth patterns of destructive moles have led many investigators to consider the invasive mole as trophoblastic new growth or to classify it as neoplasia. If the histopathogenesis of invasive mole was dependently followed by that of hydatidiform mole, the latter would be classified in the neoplastic category with invasive mole. In other words, if it could be demonstrated that invasive mole is a result of continuous changes of the hydatidiform mole, hydatidiform mole could be considered a neoplastic disease. Although it is difficult to demonstrate the change from hydatidiform mole by experimental methods, this has been attempted using various histological, cytogenetic, and clinical studies because the problem ultimately concerns the clinical field.

In a previous chromosomal study by the author and coworkers, trophoblastic diseases were extensively investigated with special regard to changes of chromosomes in relation to malignant changes in the cell. In hydatidiform moles, which are generally presumed to derive from placental villi, a chromosomal shift from diploidy to tetraploidy was frequently found. A tendency to shift from tetraploidy or diploidy to heteroploidy was a

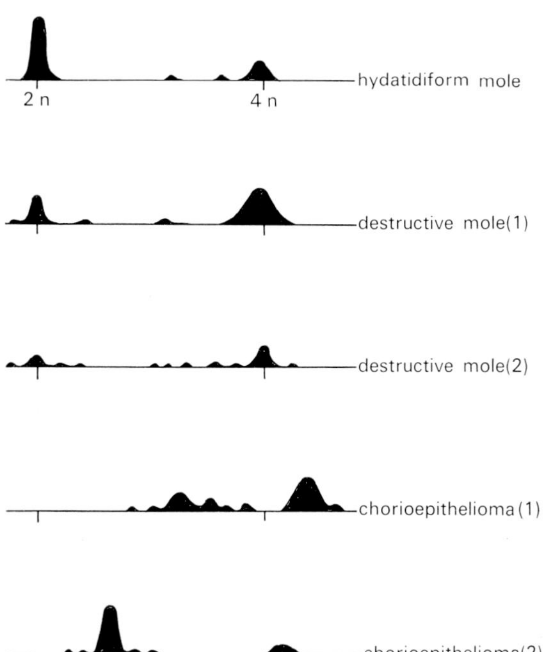

Figure 5. Diagrammatic representation of chromosome number distribution in trophoblastic tumor.

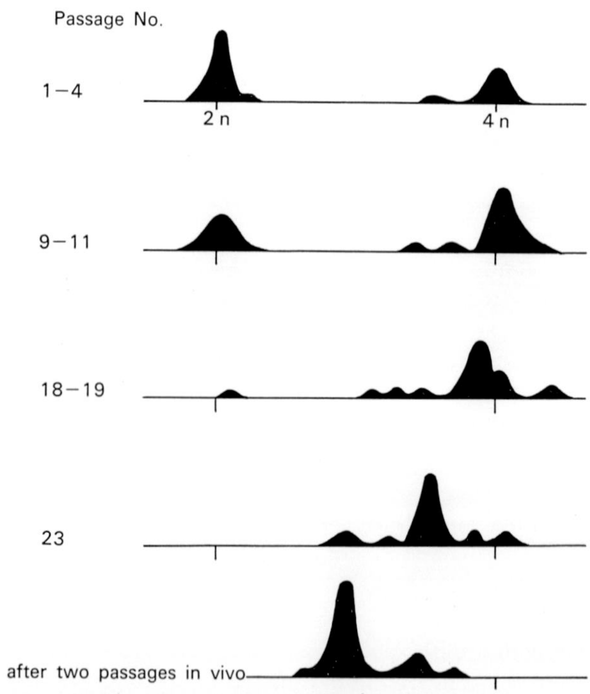

Figure 6. Schematic drawing of chromosomal role in cancerogenesis as studied in serial tissue culture of mammalian cells (Reproduced from Levan & Biesele: 1958 [1]).

notable feature of invasive moles, whereas the heteroploid cell was common in choriocarcinomas (Figure 5). These transformation patterns could be compared to those occurring in the course of the malignant transformation of mammalian cells in in vitro transfers (Figure 6) [2]. Based on the above consideration, coupled with the cytogenetic data obtained for trophoblastic disease, it may be reasonably concluded that hydatidiform mole, invasive mole, and choriocarcinoma are not of independent origin, but are mutually dependent and are successive stages of malignant transformation; also, the degree of chromosomal aberration in them tends to increase with increasing malignancy. These chromosomal findings seem to endorse the view that choriocarcinoma occurs as a result of malignant transformation following in succession from invasive mole and hydatidiform mole. The present study presents some morphological aspects of trophoblastic disease correlated with the above chromosomal findings, particularly concerning the relationship between hydatidiform mole and invasive mole.

Initially, at the time of hysterectomy or evacuation, specimens in this study were divided carefully according to the diagnostic criteria. Usually hydatidiform mole with its characteristic feature is not difficult to diagnose immediately at the time of evacuation from the uterine cavity. However, the morbid features of destructive mole within the uterine wall were diagnosed after hysterectomy by macroscopically examining the sagittal section of the uterus. Microscopical examination of the specimens was also performed, but classification was not made.

The degree of the destructive grading of the destructive mole in the myometrium was classified according to the macroscopical features as shown in Table 1 and Figure 1.

The grading of invasive mole features and the time interval between the evacuation

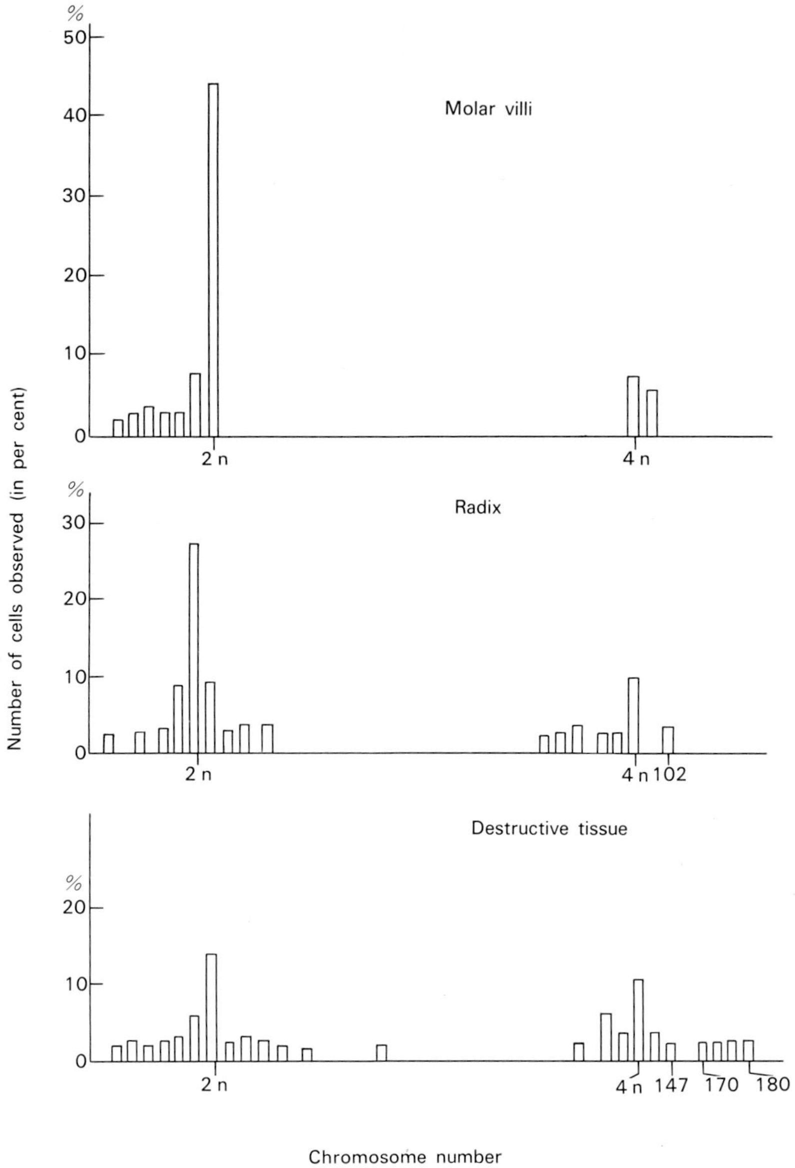

Figure 7. Distribution of chromosome number in molar villi, radix, and destructive tissue.

of hydatidiform mole and the hysterectomy demonstrating a invasive mole is presented in Figure 2. In clinical experience, it was noted that the origin of invasive mole may depend on the hydatidiform mole, as hydatidiform mole always occurs as an antecedent disease with at least a 1-week interval between the occurrence of hydatidiform mole and invasive mole (Figure 2).

The results of the above investigations indicate that the degree of the invasive mole morbidity in the uterine wall is related to the interval after evacuation of hydatidiform mole and parallel to the degree of the chromosomal aberration noted in previous studies. It also may be noted that the most prevalent types of destructive features, which occur

Table 2. Course of change of hydatidiform mole

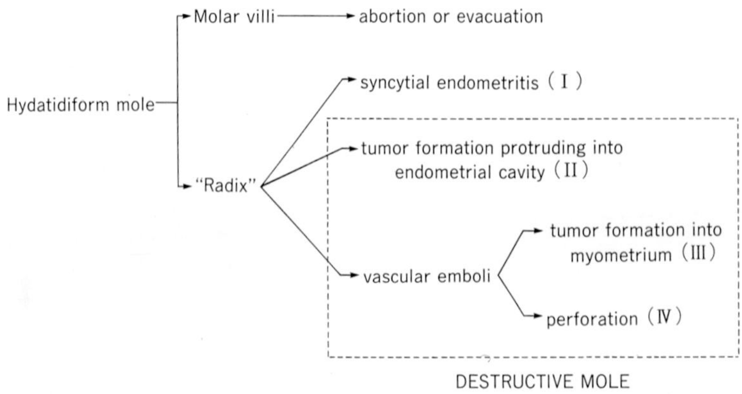

several weeks after evacuation of the mole, are elevated tumor formation in the uterine cavity (grade II) and tumor formation within the myometrium (grade III). It is very interesting that the two prevalent types of destructive features show morphological similarity to the radix of mole, and their chromosomal constitution also shows a close similarity in pattern (Figure 7). Furthermore, macroangiographical studies also indicate that the emboli type is the next most common feature, and it is frequently a combined feature of both grades III and IV (Figure 3). The perforation type (grade IV) was considered as one type of tumor formation within the myometrium. Through the above macrohistological, chromosomal, and histogenetic investigations and the clinical follow-up observation of the occurrence of invasive mole features, the courses of hydatidiform mole changes can be arranged as shown in Table 2. This macrohistological investigation and these chromosomal studies suggest the concept that the histogenesis and origin of invasive mole might be derived from the process of hydatidiform mole cell transformation toward malignancy, as has been demonstrated.

REFERENCES

1. Benirschke K, Driscoll SG: The Pathology of the Human Placenta, 1st ed. Springer-Verlag, New York, 1967, pp. 362, 364–366, 373.
2. Levan A, Biesele JJ: Role of chormosomes in carciogenesis, as studied in serial tissue culture of mammalian cells. Ann NY Acad Sci 71: 1022–1025, 1958.
3. Makino S, Sasaki MS, Fukuschima T: Cytological studies of tumors. XLI. Chromosomal instability in human chorionic lesions. Okajimas Folia Anat Jpn 40: 439–465, 1965.

PART FIVE

CHEMOTHERAPY OF TROPHOBLASTIC DISEASES

17

Twenty-Five Years' Experience In Chemotherapy of Choriocarcinoma and Invasive Mole

Song Hong-Zhao, Wu Pao-Chen, Tang Min Yi, and Yang Xiu-Yu

Comprehensive study of choriocarcinoma and invasive mole has been carried out in Capital Hospital, Peking, since 1949. In the first few years, the clinical and pathologic characteristics of these diseases were carefully studied, and a set of diagnostic methods and standards was established. However, as the method of treatment was conventional, i.e., hysterectomy with or without postoperative irradiation, the therapeutic results were very unsatisfactory. Therefore, in 1953, we began to search for some new methods of treatment. From the previous study it occurred to us that choriocarcinoma metastasized early, rapidly, and extensively, and surgery and radiotherapy were only effective for local lesions. Only drugs introduced into the body would be able to reach the pathologic lesions inaccessible to either surgery or radiotherapy. In view of this, various drugs such as nitrogen mustard, mitromin, and various herbal medicines were then tried. Through an effort sustained over several years, five chemical agents were proved effective for this group of diseases. Successful application of these drugs has significantly reduced the mortality.

Following is a brief summary of the therapeutic results during the past 25 years. Part of the work had been previously reported [1, 2].

DIAGNOSTIC CRITERIA AND CLINICAL STAGING

From 1959 through 1978, 448 cases of choriocarcinoma and 492 cases of invasive mole were admitted and treated nonselectively. On admission all patients underwent investigative studies, including chest radiography, hematology profiles, and human chorionic gonadotropin (hCG) determinations. Hysterogram, pyelogram, electrocardiogram, arteriography, heptosplenic or cerebral scan, and ultrasonography as well as computed tomography scan were performed when indicated.

For a diagnosis of choriocarcinoma, a histologic diagnosis had to have been made by examination of a sufficient number of tissue specimens showing hyperplastic and dystroplastic trophoblast without formed stromal villi, or the lesion had to have developed in association with a pregnancy in which the placenta was totally devoid of molar changes. Invasive mole was diagnosed whenever a histopathologic diagnosis was available or after evacuation of a hydatidiform mole when there was persistent trophoblastic disease as evidenced by a plateau or increase in the hCG titer and/or presence of metastasis. In this manner no cases of invasive mole were included in the choriocarcinoma group, although some cases of choriocarcinoma may have been included as invasive mole. In this series 75% of the cases were diagnosed on a pathologic basis.

The criteria of clinical staging followed those proposed by us in 1962 (presented at the Eighth International Congress of Cancer Control held in Moscow and published in *Acta UICC* in 1964 [1], as shown in Figure 1. Table 1 shows the clinical stages of the admitted patients. Metastases to different sites were revealed in 88.4% of choriocarcinoma cases and in 62.6% of invasive mole cases. About 50% of the choriocarcinoma patients were stage IIIB and stage IV, which indicates that most of the admitted patients were late cases. This is because currently most hospitals are able to treat early cases and only late or resistant cases are referred to us.

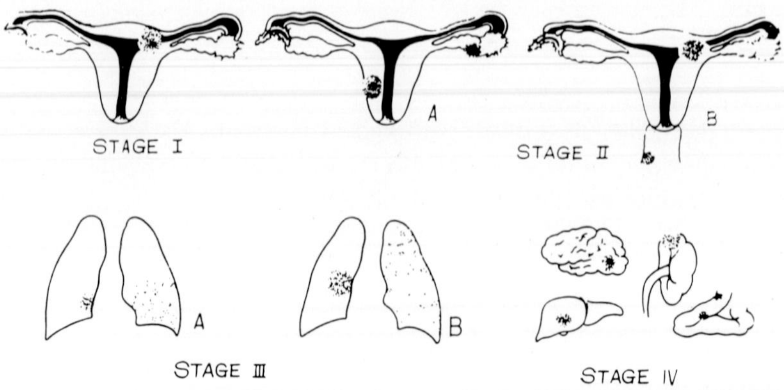

Figure 1. Criteria of clinical staging. Stage I=The lesion is limited to the uterus. Stage II=The lesion has extended outside the uterus, but is still confined to the genital organs; A: extension to parametrium or appendages; B: vaginal metastasis. Stage III=Pulmonary metastasis; A: cotton ball-like shadows not exceeding 3 cm or the area covered by patchy shadows not exceeding half the lung on one side; B: conditions exceeding the above. Stage IV=Generalized metastases to the brain, liver, kidney, spleen, intestines, skin, and so on.

Table 1. Clinical stages of admitted patients

	I (%)	II (%)	III		IV (%)	Total
			A(%)	B(%)		
Choriocarcinoma	52 (11.6)	30 (6.4)	140 (31.3)	126 (28.1)	100 (22.3)	448
Malignant mole	184 (37.4)	56 (11.4)	217 (44.1)	21 (4.3)	14 (2.8)	492

METHODS OF TREATMENT

The methods of treatment differed in different periods. During the first period (1958–1964), oral administration of large doses of 6-mercaptopurine (6MP) was used together with surgery. 5-Fluorouracil (5FU) and kengshengmycin (KSM) were the drugs of first choice in the second period (1965–1968). During the third period (1969–1972) combined administration of two or more drugs was the routine method of treatment. Two newly synthesized chemicals, tisupurine (AT1438) and nitrocaphane (AT1258) were

Table 2. Method of treatment

Chemicals used	Daily dosage	Method of administration	Course duration (day)	Interval between courses (wk)
6MP	6.0–6.5 mg/kg	By mouth in 2 divided doses	10	4
5FU	28–30 mg/kg	Dissolved in 500 mL 5% glucose, slow infusion for 8 hr	10	2
KSM	8–10 μg/kg	Dissolved in 500 mL 5% glucose, slow infusion for 4 hr	10	2
AT1438	8–12 mg/kg	Dissolved in 500 mL 5% glucose, slow infusion for 4 hr	10	3
AT1258	0.6–0.8 mg/kg	Dissolved in 20 mL saline, intravenous	10	3
MTX	10–15 mg	Dissolved in 4–6 mL distilled water, intrathoracic	Every 2–4 day; total 50 mg a course	

6MP=6-mercaptopurine; 5FU=5-fluorouracil; KSM=kengshengmycin; AT1438=tisupurine; AT1258=nitrocaphane; MTX=methotrexate.

Table 3. Specific treatment regimens for different sites of metastases

Site of metastasis [Ref.]	Specific treatment regimen
Vulval and/or vaginal metastasis	When there is no ulceration or bleeding, intravenous infusion with 5FU alone or in combination with KSM usually results in rapid resolution of metastasis. In case of bleeding, vaginal packing is used. Local injection of 5FU is rarely needed.
Parametrial or pelvic metastasis	Intravenous infusion of 5FU+KSM is usually effective. If not, local injection or intraarterial infusion (through catheterization of the femoral artery) of 5FU may be useful. In resistant cases pelvic irradiation may be added.
Pulmonary metastasis [4]	5FU+KSM intravenous infusion or KSM+AT1258 may be used. If complicated by hemothorax, intrathoracic injection of 5FU after tapping may be given. Lobectomy may be selectively done in drug-resistant cases.
Cerebral metastasis [3]	A triple protocol is adopted: 1) 5FU+KSM intravenous infusion to control the accompanied pulmonary or other metastasis; 2) intrathecal injection of MTX or intraarterial infusion of 5FU or 6MP (through catheterization of the internal carotid artery) to control the local lesion; 3) symptomatic treatment to reduce the increased intracranial pressure, to control convulsions, to relieve severe headache, etc. Surgical removal of the lesion or whole-brain irradiation may be tried in resistant cases.
Hepatic metastasis	Intravenous infusion of 5FU+KSM is usually effective. If not, oral administration or intraarterial infusion (through catheterization of the hepatic artery) of 5FU may be added.
Splenic, renal, or intestinal metastasis	5FU+KSM intravenous drip is effective. Surgery is needed when profuse bleeding endangers the life of the patient.

Abbreviation as in Table 2.

found to be effective and were used in combination therapy when indicated. During the last period (1976–1978) specific treatment schedules were designed for different sites of metastases. Methotrexate (MTX) was used only occasionally for the treatment of cerebral metastasis since 1962.

The dosage and methods of administration of these drugs are listed in Table 2, and the specific schedules for different sites of metastasis are listed in Table 3. The treatment was continued until complete remission was achieved. Then one or more courses were given for consolidation before discharge. No maintenance treatment was given.

Since 1968 surgery has been performed only occasionally. Hysterectomy, splenectomy, or nephrectomy was done when profuse bleeding endangered the life of the patient, and lobectomy was practiced in cases with pulmonary metastases resistant to chemotherapy. In a few cases, craniotomy for removal of cerebral lesions was tried when medical treatment failed to give satisfactory results. Chemotherapy was given for 2 to 3 days before surgical intervention and was continued postoperatively until a regular course was completed.

RESULTS OF TREATMENT

From 1959 to 1978, a total of 940 cases of gestational trophoblastic diseases (consisting of 448 cases of choriocarcinoma and 492 cases of invasive mole) were treated nonselectively. The results of treatment compared with that before 1958 are shown in Table 4. The mortality of choriocarcinoma was reduced from 89.2% before 1958 to 17.8% during the last period (1976–1978) and that of invasive mole from 25.9% to 1.3%.

The therapeutic results in choriocarcinoma according to clinical staging is shown in Figure 2. The mortalities for stage I and stage II in the last period were nil. For stage IIIA the mortality was reduced from 100% to around 6%. However, the results of treatment in stage IIIB and stage IV were still unsatisfactory. The mortalities were 25.0% and 38.5%, respectively. The overall mortality of metastatic choriocarcinoma during the last period was 20.1%.

The metastatic sites in 35 cases of choriocarcinoma and 11 cases of invasive mole who recovered from stage IV disease are shown in Table 5. In one case of choriocarcinoma, there were metastases to eight organs, including brain, lung, liver, spleen, left kidney, gastrointestinal tract, scalp, and both ovaries. The patient was cured and has survived for 15 years up to present. Table 6 shows the therapeutic results in brain and liver metastases.

Since 1959, there have been 208 patients who were treated by chemotherapy alone in order to preserve reproductive function. A total of 322 pregnancies occurred in 183 patients, with 271 live births (four twins). There was no increase of recurrence of the disease nor obstetrical complications. All the children grew normally, except for six neonatal deaths including two malformations. The oldest child is now 23 years old. The details are recorded in Table 7.

All the survivors were followed up periodically. The durations of survival are shown in Table 8. All of them were followed up for at least 5 years. About 75% were followed up for more than 10 years about 50% were followed up for more than 15 years, with 95 cases being followed up more than 20 years. Repeated examinations with hCG radioimmunoassay and chest x-ray revealed no evidence of residual or recurrent disease, which indicated cure.

The therapeutic efficacy of different drugs when used alone as the primary treatment

Table 4. Therapeutic results (mortality) during different periods*

Periods	Methods of treatment	Choriocarcinoma			Malignant mole			Total		
		Cases	Deaths	%	Cases	Deaths	%	Cases	Deaths	%
1949–1958	Surgery with or without irradiation	37	33	89.2	27	7	25.9	64	40	62.5
1959–1964	6MP with surgery	109	67	61.5	78	14	17.9	187	81	43.3
1965–1968	5FU or KSM	149	57	38.3	182	11	6.0	331	68	20.5
1969–1972	Multidrugs, multiroutes	78	26	33.3	82	0	0	160	26	16.3
1973–1975	Specific regimens for different metastases	56	12	21.4	72	1	1.4	128	13	10.2
1976–1978	Specific regimens for different metastases	56	10	17.8	78	1	1.3	134	11	8.2

* Of all deaths, 20 cases were due to drug toxicity, 5 cases were due to causes not related to this disease, and 10 cases were lost to follow-up and were considered as deaths.

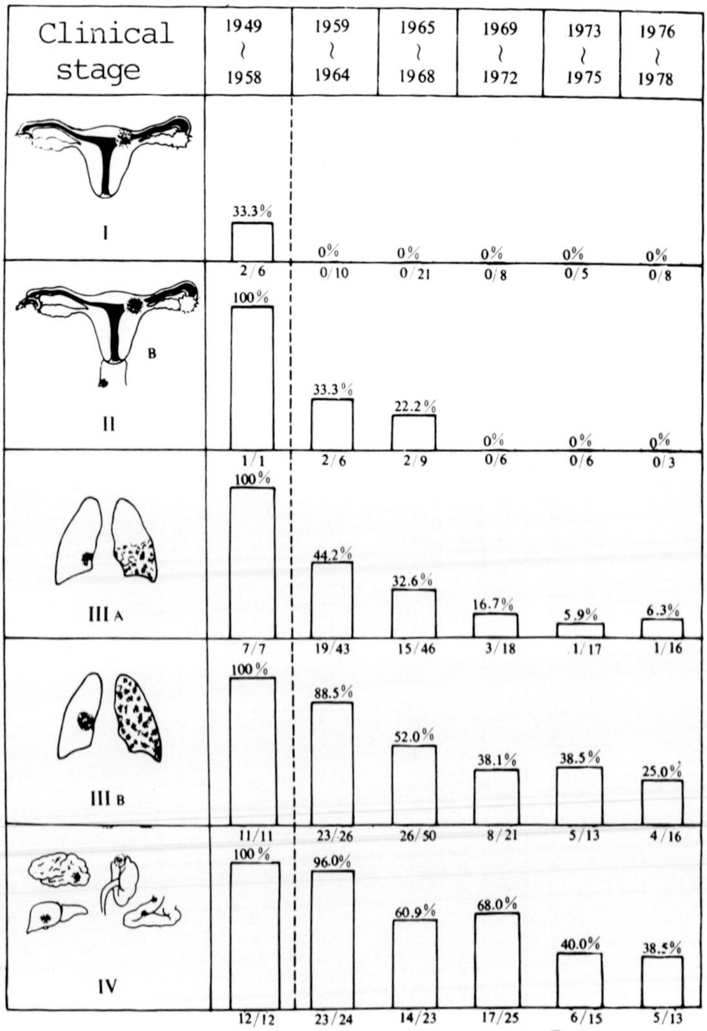

Figure 2. Therapeutic results of choriocarcinoma at different stages in different periods.

Table 5. Sites of metastases in 46 cases recovered from stage IV disease

Sites of metastasis	Choriocarcinoma (n=35)	Invasive mole (n=11)
Lung	35	11
Brain	27	6
Spinal cord	3	0
Liver	12	0
Spleen	10	0
Kidneys and/or bladder	8	0
Intestines	5	0
Skin and/or muscle	4	0

was evaluated. The results are shown in Table 9. The toxic reactions to different drugs are shown in Tables 10 and 11. Among the 940 patients treated, there were 20 deaths directly or indirectly related to drug toxicity. Most of the deaths occurred in the early part of this study (Table 12).

Table 6. Therapeutic results (mortality) in brain and liver metastases

Period	Brain metastasis			Liver metastasis		
	No. of cases treated	Deaths	%	No. of cases treated	Deaths	%
1949–1958	12	12	100.0	12	12	100.0
1959–1964	33	31	93.9	16	16	100.0
1965–1968	32	27	84.4	8	6	75.0
1969–1972	20	13	65.0	8	5	62.5
1973–1975	13	6	46.1	4	1	25.0
1976–1978	9	3	33.3	6	2	33.3

Table 7. Subsequent pregnancy after recovery (through 1983)

	Choriocarcinoma	Invasive mole	Total
Total patients	28	180	208
Patients pregnant	22 (78.6%)	161 (89.4%)	183
Total pregnancies	40	282	322
Abortion	0	22	22
Miscarriage	7	20	27
Ectopic	2	0	2
Stillbirth	1	1	2
Death in utero	0	2	2
Live birth	30	241*	271*
Neonatal death	1	3	4
Malformations	0	2	2
Total no. of living children	29	236	265
Age of living children			
5 yr	5	29	34
5–9 yr	13	77	90
10–14 yr	1	88	99
15–19 yr	0	38	38
20 yr	0	4	4

* Twins.

Table 8. Duration of survival (through 1983)

	No. of cases	>5 yr	>10 yr	>15 yr	>20 yr
Choriocarcinoma	276	276 (100.0%)	199 (72.1%)	134 (48.6%)	31 (11.2%)
Invasive mole	465	465 (100.0%)	346 (74.4%)	235 (50.5%)	64 (13.8%)
Total	741	741 (100.0%)	545 (73.5%)	369 (49.8%)	95 (12.8%)

Table 9. Therapeutic efficacy of different drugs initially used

		6MP	5FU	KSM	AT1438
Choriocarcinoma	No. of cases treated	98	86	44	7
	No. of complete remissions	46	51	22	3
	% remissions	46.9	59.3	50.0	42.9
Invasive mole	No. of cases treated	61	126	78	3
	No. of complete remissicns	51	107	51	2
	% remissions	83.6	84.9	65.4	66.7
Total	No. of cases treated	159	212	122	10
	No. of complete remissions	97	158	73	5
	% remissions	61.0	74.5	59.8	50.0

Abbreviations as in Table 2.

Table 10. Effect of different drugs on blood count

Drugs (medication courses)	White blood cells—lowest value (1,000/mm³)					Platelets—lowest value (10,000/mm³)				
	<1	1–2	2–3	3–4	>4	<1	1–3	3–5	5–10	>10
6MP (138)	5.1	31.2	47.2	10.1	6.5 (%)	8.0	34.0	26.1	24.6	7.2 (%)
AT1438 (33)	2.7	27.1	48.6	16.2	5.4 (%)	10.8	13.5	18.9	32.5	24.3 (%)
5FU (950)	0.7	4.1	10.8	18.4	65.9 (%)	0.5	3.7	6.0	31.2	58.6 (%)
KSM (402)	0.2	0.7	4.0	8.2	86.8 (%)	0.5	7.7	8.0	29.4	54.5 (%)
5FU+KSM (139)	0	30.8	17.9	12.8	38.5 (%)	3.6	12.6	20.5	28.2	35.9 (%)
MTX (66)	9.1	30.4	30.4	15.1	15.1 (%)	7.6	28.8	22.7	30.9	10.6 (%)

Abbreviations as in Table 2.

Table 11. Effect of different drugs on liver functions

Drugs (medication courses)	SGPT elevated %
6MP (138)	42.7
MTX (66)	23.0
KSM (360)	15.0
5FU (749)	6.4

SGPT=serum glutamic-pyruvic transaminase.
Other abbreviations as in Table 2.

Table 12. Deaths related to drug toxicity

Period	No. of cases treated	Deaths	%
1959–1964	187	13	6.9
1965–1968	331	4	1.2
1969–1972	160	2	1.25
1973–1975	128	1	0.8
1976–1978	134	0	0

COMMENTS

The first drug that we used with success in the treatment of choriocarcinoma and invasive mole was 6MP. During the course of an investigation of contraceptive drugs, 6MP was found to have strong embryocidal activity. As trophoblastic tumors are embryonic in origin, it occurred to us that this agent might be effective in the treatment of this group of diseases. Therefore, trials were made in 1958. In the beginning, the conventional dosage for leukemia was tried. The patient died before the completion of a course of medication, but pathologic examinations of autopsy material revealed distinct effect of the drug on tumor cells. New trials were then made by gradually increasing the daily doses and shortening the duration of a course. When the drug dose was increased to 2.5 times the dosage for leukemia, good response was obtained. On this regimen a case of choriocarcinoma with pulmonary metastasis was discharged in complete remission from this hospital for the first time. The same regimen was also effective in invasive mole. The mortalities in this group of diseases have shown a marked decrease since then.

However, on further investigation, it was found that a number of cases did not respond well to 6MP either initially or after several courses of treatment. To save the lives of these patients, new trials were carried out to search for more effective agents. As 5FU and 6MP both belonged to the same antimetabolite group, the former was then put into clinical trial. At first, intravenous injection of the conventional dosage of 5FU was used. Patients could not tolerate a complete course of 10 days because of toxicity. Later, by diluting 5FU with 500 mL of 5% dextrose and giving it by intravenous infusion slowly, toxic reactions were markedly reduced. This provided a possibility of increasing the dosage without increasing the toxicity. When the daily dosage was increased to nearly twice the conventional one, it was found that this chemical had a better therapeutic effect and less toxicity than 6MP. It has been used as the drug of choice since 1965.

Following the successful use of these two agents, several others such as kengshengmycin (KSM), tisupurine (AT1438), and nitrocaphane (AT1258) were also found. Kengshengmycin is a new antibiotic obtained from a strain of Streptomycetes isolated from the soil of the southern part of China. Chemically it is similar but not identical to actinomycin D. Tisupurine is a water-solube derivative of 6MP and has same action as the parent compound with a less toxic reaction. Nitrocaphane is a new derivative of sarcolysin. These agents were added to the list of drugs for the treatment of choriocarcinoma and its allied diseases. As the number of effective drugs increased, various combinations of these drugs were studied. Some proved to have better effects, and have been used routinely since 1969.

Experience over years of clinical practice has uncovered the fact that though these agents are all effective against choriocarcinoma, they have differing degrees of effectiveness at different sites of metastasis and by different routes of administration. For instance, 5FU is more effective for metastases to the genitourinary and digestive tract, whereas KSM is more effective in pulmonary metastasis. When 5FU was used for pulmonary metastasis, intravenous infusion produced better therapeutic results than administration through other routes. Therefore, a specific treatment regimen was designed for each site of metastasis. This again greatly improved the therapeutic results.

Among all these drugs, due emphasis should be given to 5FU. It possesses several merits superior to others. First, 5FU has a wide range of effectiveness for different sites of metastasis, such as metastases to the lungs, liver, gastrointestinal tract, and genitourinary system. Second, when diluted with 500 mL 5% glucose and given slowly through intravenous drip for 8 hours, 5FU causes the least number and degree of toxic reactions of any drug so far in our experience. Third, 5FU may be given through various routes, such as the intraarterial, intravenous, intraperitoneal, and intrathoracic as well as directly into the tumor mass. It may also be given by mouth. Such a very wide range of routes of administration facilitates our selection of it to treat different sites of metastasis. Because of these merits, 5FU has become the drug of first choice in our practice.

To ensure the therapeutic effect and to avoid severe toxic reaction, several points must be carefully observed. The therapeutic effect and toxic reactions of 5FU are clossly related to dosage and method of administration. The dosage given in this report was formulated through repeated trials and should not be changed without apparent reasons. Daily dose less than 25 mg/kg will weaken therapeutic effect, and daily dose greater than 30 mg/kg will enhance the toxic reaction. But, if the patient has a body weight greater than 60 kg, the dose should be reduced: the total daily dosage of 5FU should not exceed 1750 mg. In this case, 5FU should be used in combination with other effective agents.

The speed of administration of 5FU is another matter of crucial importance. Long-term clinical practice has proved optimal a duration of 8 hours for a given dose of 5FU dissolved in 500 mL of 5% dextrose evenly instilled into the patient. If the 5FU-dextrose solution is given too quickly, e.g., in less than 4 hours, the toxic reaction will be very much augmented; if given too slowly the therapeutic effect will be inconspicuous.

The third important point is the special toxic reaction of 5FU: diarrhea that may sometimes result in pseudomembranous colitis if not properly managed. This is a very dreadful complication and should be watched carefully. Once diarrhea occurs during chemotherapy with 5FU, the medication should be withdrawn immediately, and the frequency of the bowel movement and the character of the stools should be watched constantly. For the early detection of this disease, it is necessary to monitor the bacterial flora in the smear of fecal materials. When Gram-positive bacilli (*Clostridium difficile*) and cocci (*Staphylococcus aureus*) become dominant and pseudomembranous colitis is strongly suspected, appropriate treatment with vancomycin and metronidazole should be given as soon as possible.

REFERENCES

1. Sung HC, Wu PC, Ho JH: The treatment of choriocarcinoma and chorioadenoma destruens with 6MP and surgery. In Chinese Academy of Medical Sciences (eds): Selected Papers on Cancer Research. Shanghai Sci Tech Publ, Shanghai, 1962, pp. 441–451. Republished in Acta Unio Internationalis Contra Cancerum 20: 491–502, 1964.
2. Sung HC, et al.: Cure of choriocarcinoma and chorioadenoma destruens by chemotherapy. Sci Sin 26: 298–316, 1973.
3. Sung HC, Wu P-C: Brain metastasis of choriocarcinoma and malignant mole: Its clinical course, diagnosis and treatment. Chin Med J 92: 164–174, 1979.
4. Wang YE, Sung HC, Sun CF, et al.: Drug resistant pulmonary metastasis of choriocarcinoma, treated by lobectomy (report of 29 cases). Chin Med J 93: 758–766, 1980.

18

Progress in the Chemotherapy of Choriocarcinoma

K. D. Bagshawe, R. H. J. Begent, E. S. Newlands, and G. J. S. Rustin

There have been many advances in the chemotherapy of choriocarcinoma in the 30 years since the first reports of the use of chemotherapeutic agents. At the same time this use has introduced several new problems. This paper reviews our experience at Charing Cross Hopital in London, but does not attempt to review the work of other groups. Many of the most difficult cases that we have seen in recent years were referred from Europe and the Middle East, often after prolonged and unsuccessful chemotherapy.

As most trophoblastic tumors are now eradicable and about 40% of our patients are childless, hysterectomy is undesirable as a means of obtaining a histological diagnosis. As a result, it is neither necessary nor practicable to make a distinction between invasive mole and choriocarcinoma in all cases. After a woman has a hydatidiform mole persisting trophoblastic activity is detected by the presence of human chorionic gonadotropin (hCG) in serum, and often there are persisting abnormalities detected in the uterine pattern by ultrasound examination. In our experience, however, these do not distinguish invasive mole from choriocarcinoma and curettage rarely provides tissue that allows a decisive histological diagnosis. Statistically, the probability that a postmole trophoblastic proliferation is choriocarcinoma increases with length of time after evacuation. In any case, the distinction in the early postmole period may be academic, and chemotherapeutic failures have now been virtually eliminated in this group.

In this series there have been no deaths from invasive mole. Furthermore, all cases following nonmole pregnancies for whom adequate material was available for histological examination have proved to be choriocarcinoma, with the exception of a small group of patients now recognized to have had placental site tumor.

PLACENTAL SITE TUMOR

Placental site tumor is a rare form of gestational trophoblastic neoplasm that appears to have several features distinguishing it from choriocarcinoma [7, 9]. It appears to arise predominantly from nonmole pregnancy. Histologically it consists of relatively uniform fields of cytotrophoblastic cells with less syncytium formation than in choriocarcinoma. The reduced amount of syncytium may account for the finding that few cells stain for hCG, but many cells stain for human placental lactogen (hPL) and also stain with a recently described cytotrophoblastic monoclonal antibody [10]. The serum hCG values tend to be much lower than those associated with a similar body burden of choriocarcinoma. An additional distinctive feature may be the occurrence in some patients of nephrotic syndrome—edema, proteinuria, and hypertension. Our experience with cases having this syndrome is that it was reversed in two cases by hysterectomy. The most important reason for distinguishing this rare tumor from choriocarcinoma is that its response to cytotoxic agents is limited. If this tumor is detected, hysterectomy should be performed at an early stage in the hope of preventing the development of metastases. It is possible that some of the therapeutic failures in our series of "choriocarcinomas" between 1958 and 1980 were unrecognized examples of placental site tumor.

RETROSPECTIVE ANALYSIS OF CAUSES OF DEATH

Between 1958 and 1982 a total of 860 patients were treated by chemotherapy for invasive mole or choriocarcinoma; 109 of these patients died. There were two principal causes of death, which we define as early and late causes.

EARLY CAUSES OF DEATH

Of the 109 deaths, 26 occurred in the first month of treatment, and most of these were in the first 2 weeks. These early causes of death were attributable to the initial extent of disease or to metastases in specific anatomical sites. The sites of importance are lung, liver, brain, and gastrointestinal tract. The problem arises also from the fact that when tumors are first exposed to intense cytotoxic action, physical changes perhaps of an edematous nature take place and may convert a critical situation into a fatal one.

Although pulmonary metastases tend to be silent, the situation changes if they become extensive and confluent. Dyspnea and cyanosis may then be present at rest or on slight exertion. During the first few days of chemotherapy in such patients, there appears to be a fall in arterial O_2 tension and a loss of pulmonary compliance, so respiratory failure may ensue. This is sometimes referred to as tumor lysis syndrome, although it is by no means clear what mechanisms are involved.

Patients with liver metastases may suffer intrahepatic or intraabdominal hemorrhage. Brain metastases may undergo edematous change with increase in intracranial pressure or hemorrhage.

In all these situations it seems important that the first course of chemotherapy and possibly the second course should be given at reduced dosages to minimize the risks. Respiratory assistance should be introduced early. In the case of brain metastases it may be appropriate to alert the neurosurgical team, as well as to make use of dexamethasone and possibly diuretics to control intracranial pressure.

In the case of metastases in the gastrointestinal tract, it is important to recognize that these may be multiple and very small; therefore resection should not be attempted. They may also be large and even grow through the anterior abdominal wall, producing fecal fistulas. These lesions all seem capable of resolution with judicious chemotherapy, transfusions, antibiotics, and careful nursing.

The use of reduced chemotherapeutic dosages is, of course, also necessary in patients with impaired renal or hepatic function. When using reduced dose levels care must be taken not to increase the risk of drug resistance at a later stage in therapy. Full dosage should be used as soon as the patient's general condition permits.

LATE CAUSES OF DEATH

Of the 109 deaths in the series, 75 occurred after chemotherapy had been in progress for many months. These were attributable to drug resistance. All but two of the six drug-induced "toxic" deaths were related to the intensification of chemotherapy in response to drug resistance.

The avoidance of drug resistance has been a major objective from the start of these studies. It is still not widely known that very few, if any, advanced cases of choriocarcinomas are completely eradicated by methotrexate alone.

Our earliest attempt to avoid drug resistance was the use of 6-mercaptopurine with methotrexate. This appeared to be much more effective than methotrexate alone [4]. Although 6-mercaptopurine is only a weak antitrophoblastic agent, good use of it has been made of it in China [16]. Combination of actinomycin-D and methotrexate was found to cause substantial mucositis. In 1963 we found that methotrexate with folinic acid (leucovorin) was effective and nontoxic in many cases. This became our standard initial therapy for several years [5]. When patients became resistant, other drugs were then introduced. Subsequent analysis showed that although this approach was very satisfactory for many patients, there were also many failures. In some patients resistance to methotrexate appeared to confer resistance to other drugs. It was clear that there was a broad spectrum of heterogeneity in trophoblastic neoplasms, some of which responded readily and others only with great difficulty.

A total of 317 patients treated between 1958 and 1973 were analyzed for factors that might indicate the propensity of the tumor for drug resistance [2]. Twelve prognostic factors were identified, and numerical scores were assigned for each of these. A total prognostic score was obtained for each patient by adding the scores for each factor. Low-scoring patients all survived, whereas those with the highest scores all died. A somewhat simpler scoring system, which eliminates factors that cannot be obtained for all patients, was published subsequently by WHO [8].

This prognostic score is therefore an indication of the probability that the tumor will become resistant with a sequential introduction of cytotoxic agents. The fact that there were many deaths in the high-scoring group raised the question of whether it would be advantageous to introduce all the known effective agents early in treatment. On this basis we have stratified our treatment protocols at three levels for low, middle, and high risk.

LOW-RISK PATIENTS

These are patients scoring up to 5 on the WHO prognostic scale [8] (or scoring less than 50 on the earlier scale [2]). In our series, 405 patients have been treated in this risk category between 1958 and 1983. The only death was from pneumonia during an influenza epidemic. Virtually all these patients were treated with our methotrexate/folinic acid regimen (Table 1). However, approximately 30% required additional therapy with other drugs, either to achieve complete remission or accelerate attainment of remission. Treatment was given during alternating weeks and continued until hCG was undetectable (i.e., <2 IU/liter) for 6 weeks.

MIDDLE-RISK PATIENTS

These patients scored 6 to 9 on the WHO scale (a score of 60 to 90 on the earlier scale). They have been treated since 1974 with a protocol that provides single drugs or simple drug combinations in quick succession, e.g., courses A, B, C, D, A, B, etc. (Table 2). Retaining this pattern of drug administration has been valuable for the purpose of identifying new agents effective against choriocarcinoma. This led to the identification of VP16213 (etoposide) as a powerful drug for choriocarcinoma in 1977 [11].

Between 1958 and 1983 there were 232 patients in this category. Three of them died from drug resistance despite the use of all effective agents. There have been no deaths in this group since the introduction of etoposide. Treatment in this group is generally continued until hCG has been undetectable for 8 to 10 weeks.

Table 1. Low-risk regimen

Methotrexate 50 mg (or 1 mg/kg with maximum 70 mg) by intramuscular injection every 48 hours ×4
Folinic acid (leucovorin, calcium folinate) 6 mg 30 hours after each injection of methotrexate by intramuscular injection or by mouth
Courses start: day 1, 14, 28, etc.

Table 2. Middle-risk regimen

Course A
Etoposide (VP16-213) 100 mg/m^2 in 200 mL saline by intravenous infusion over 30 minutes, daily for 5 consecutive days
Course B
Day 1. Hydroxyurea (hydroxycarbamide) 0.5 g repeated after 12 hours by mouth
Days 2–8. Methotrexate and folinic acid (as in Table 1) plus 6-mercaptopurine 75 mg daily on folinic acid days only
Course C
Actinomycin-D (dactinomycin) 0.5 mg (or 10 to 12 μg/kg) intravenously daily for 5 days.
Course D
Vincristine (Oncovin) 1 mg/m^2 on days 1 and 3; cyclophosphamide (Cytoxan) 400 mg/m^2 intravenously on days 1 and 3

The sequence of courses is A, B, C, D, A, B, etc., or regimen D may be held in reserve in case one course proves toxic or ineffective. The sequence then would be A, B, C, A, B, etc.

The interval between the end of a course and the start of the next should not be more than 7 days unless there is persisting toxicity, but should not be greater than 10 days unless toxicity is marked.

HIGH-RISK PATIENTS

The patients in this group all had scores of 10 or more (scores of less than 100 on the earlier scale). Following the prognostic analysis, in the mid-1970s we introduced a protocol initially known as CHAMOMA that included melphalan. This was later replaced by CHAMOCA (cyclophosphamide replaced melphalan). The principle of the regimen was to combine all known effective agents in a protocol that would incur toxicity but, it was hoped, would minimize the emergence of drug resistance. Toxicity proved to be variable but was high in some patients, necessitating a recovery period between courses of treatment. This period was rarely less than 10 days and some times as much as 20 days.

Following this we retained many of the features of CHAMOCA in a new protocol, EMA-CO (Table 3). EMA-CO differs from CHAMOCA in two important respects. First, it introduces etoposide. Second, it provides treatment on a weekly basis. Also, the patient requires hospitalization for only one night every 2 weeks. Although the total drug dosage over a period of time is higher than with CNAMOCA, it is much better tolerated.

Between 1958 and 1983, there were 223 patients in the high-risk category; 105 of them died. With CHAMOCA alone, for the high-risk group the survival rate was 75%. When a 5-day course of etoposide was given alternately with CHAMOCA, this rate improved to 83%. EMA-CO gives a similar survival rate of 83% at a much lower cost in toxicity. Treatment in this category is generally continued for 11 to 13 weeks after hCG has been undetectable (i.e., $<$ 1 to 2 IU/liter).

The extension of therapy well beyond normalization of hCG values is an important factor in successful therapy. hCG at the 1.0 IU/liter level in serum corresponded with the estimated presence of some 10^4 to 10^5 trophoblastic tumor cells in earlier studies.

Patients who become resistant to EMA-CO receive an alternative regimen. The response to cisplatin is assessed in a combination with vincristine and methotrexate (methotrexate and cisplatin on different days) [12] or with vincristine, methotrexate, and bleomycin (POMB). We avoid using cisplatin as a first agent because we do not yet know its long-term effects on fertility and because it may be useful to hold at least one potentially powerful drug in reserve.

Table 3. High-risk regimen

Course A—EMA	
Day 1.	Etoposide (VP16-213) 100 mg/m^2 by intravenous infusion in 200 mL saline over 30 minutes; dactinomycin 0.5 mg intravenously immediately; methotrexate 100 mg/m^2 intravenously immediately; methotrexate 200 mg/m^2 by intravenous infusion, 12 hours
Day 2.	Etoposide 100 mg/m^2 by intravenous infusion in 200 mL saline over 30 minutes; dactinomycin 0.5 mg intravenously immediately; folinic acid (leucovorin, calcium folinate) 15 mg intramuscularly or orally every 12 hours for 4 doses beginning 24 hours after starting methotrexate
Course B—CO	
Day 8.	Vincristine (Oncovin) 1.0 mg/m^2 intravenously immediately; cyclophosphamide 600 mg/m^2 intravenously in saline

These courses should be given on days 1 and 2, 8, 15 and 16, etc. The intervals should not be extended without cause.

CENTRAL NERVOUS SYSTEM METASTASES

Even in the early 1960s there were patients who presented with brain metastases who survived. But until the late 1970s, patients who developed brain metastases during treatment all died. We have made use of serum/cerebrospinal fluid ratios of hCG, as well as computed tomography (CT) scans, to detect central nervous system disease [3, 13].

We attach great importance to, first, the detection of brain metastases at the outset of therapy and, second, the prevention of brain metastases in the course of chemotherapy. As long as there is a viable tumor in the lung, the patient is at risk for developing brain deposits. Established disease in the central nervous system is treated by increased systemic methotrexate dosage (1 g/m^2 in the EMA-CO protocol). Provided there is no evidence of increased intracranial pressure, methotrexate (10 mg) is given intrathecally at the time of systemic CO (cyclophosphamide and vincristine sulfate [Oncovin]). Prophylactic therapy is essentially the same as the central nervous system therapeutic regimen except that the standard dose of methotrexate in the EMA protocol is used and intrathecal methotrexate is given in the same way with each CO protocol.

Central nervous system metastases occurring late during chemotherapy have been successfully treated in recent years with surgery and chemotherapy [1]. Despite these measures a small number of patients still develop drug-resistant disease. As already mentioned, it is important to determine whether the tumor is placental site in type.

Patients with minimal persistent hCG value elevations are examined for sites of residual disease with a view to surgery. If results of conventional radiology, CT scan, and MRI scan are normal, immunoscintigraphy is used to try to locate residual tumor using anti-hCG labeled with ^{131}I [6]. In about a half of these drug-resistant patients, disease sites have been identified and surgical resections have achieved sustained remission. Hysterectomy is not usually undertaken unless there is evidence of resistant disease in the uterus.

Follow-up has been maintained for more than 95% of the patients that are residents of the United Kingdom. Recent analyses indicate no significant increase in infertility, congenital abnormalities in subsequent children [15], or second malignancies [14].

SUMMARY

Patients requiring chemotherapy for invasive mole or choriocarcinoma present a broad spectrum of disease. Although the majority of these patients can be assessed by a uniform body of criteria, it is important to identify and exclude from this group patients with placental site trophoblastic tumor. This rare form of trophoblastic tumor is distinctive in terms of histology, marker production, and response to chemotherapy.

Analysis of our series has shown that about 25% of all deaths resulted from complications of the extent or localization of metastatic disease at the time of diagnosis. Some of these deaths may be preventable by special precautions during the early stages of therapy.

However, the majority of deaths resulted from drug resistance. A prognostic scoring system has provided an assessment of the potential for drug resistance in each patient. In conjunction with this, a three-tier stratification has been adopted. This provides nontoxic therapy for low-risk patients and multidrug protocols for middle- and high-risk groups. Initial surgical intervention has been kept to a minimum. Deaths in the low- and middle-risk groups have been low ($<1\%$), and the majority of deaths have occurred in the high-risk category. The long-term survival rate in the high-risk group in recent years has been more than 80%.

Retrospective analysis indicated that for patients with high risk of developing drug resistance it was more effective to use multiple agents in the initial stages of therapy, rather than to introduce the drugs sequentially as resistance developed. However, we have preferred to hold cisplatin in reserve for cases resistant to the EMA-CO protocol.

Brain metastases at presentation have generally proved responsive to chemotherapy, whereas those occurring in the course of chemotherapy tended to be resistant. Surgical intervention has played an increasing role in late recurring brain metastases and in the management of residual resistant disease or recurring disease at other sites.

Immunoscintigraphy plays a useful part in locating sites of resistant disease in some patients.

There is no evidence of impairment of fertility in our choriocarcinoma patients following chemotherapy, nor is there any evidence thus far of increased risk of second malignancies in these patients.

REFERENCES

1. Athanassiou A, Begent RHJ, Newlands ES, et al.: Central nervous system metastases of choriocarcinoma. Cancer 52: 1728–1735, 1983.
2. Bagshawe KD: Risk and prognostic factors in trophoblastic neoplasia. Cancer 38: 1373–1385, 1976.
3. Bagshawe KD, Harland S: Immunodiagnosis and monitoring of gonadotrophin-producing metastases in the central nervous system. Cancer 38: 112–118, 1976.
4. Bagshawe KD, McDonald J: Treatment of choriocarcinoma with a combination of cytotoxic drugs. Br Med J 11: 426–431, 1960.
5. Bagshawe KD, Wilde CE: Infusion therapy in pelvic trophoblastic tumours. J Obstet Gynaecol Br Commw 72: 59–64, 1963.
6. Begent RHJ, Stanway G, Searle F, et al.: Radioimmunolocalisation of tumours by external scintigraphy after administration of ^{131}I antibody to human chorionic gonadotrophin. J R Soc Med 73: 624–630, 1980.
7. Eckstein RP, Paradinas FJ, Bagshawe KD: Placental site trophoblastic tumour. Histopathology 6: 211–226, 1982.
8. Report of WHO Scientific Group: Gestational trophoblastic diseases. World Health Organisation, Geneva. Technical Report Series 692, p. 51.
9. Kurman RJ, Scully RE, Norvis HJ: Trophoblastic pseudotumor of the uterus. Cancer 38: 1214–1226, 1976.
10. Loke YW, Day S, Butterworth B, et al.: Monoclonal antibody to human cytotrophoblast cross reacts with basal layers of some fetal epithelial surfaces. Placenta 5: 199–204, 1984.
11. Newlands ES, Bagshawe KD: Epipodophyllin derivative (VP16-213) in malignant teratomas and choriocarcinomas. Lancet ii: 87, 1977.
12. Newlands ES, Bagshawe KD: Activity of high dose cis-platinum in combination with vincristine and methotrexate in drug resistant choriocarcinoma. Br J Cancer 40: 943–945, 1979.
13. Rushworth AGJ, Orr AH, Bagshawe KD: The concentration of HCG in the plasma and spinal fluid of patients with trophoblastic tumours in the central nervous system. Br J Cancer 22: 253–257, 1968.
14. Rustin GJS, Rustin F, Dent J, et al.: No increase in second tumors after cytotoxic chemotherapy for gestational trophoblastic tumors. N Engl J Med 308: 473–476, 1983.
15. Rustin GJS, Booth M, Dent J, et al.:Pregnancy after cytotoxic chemotherapy for gestational trophoblastic tumors. Br Med J 288: 103–106, 1984.
16. Sung HC, Wu PC, Ho TH: Treatment of choriocarcinoma and chorioadenoma destruens with 6-mercaptopurine and surgery: A clinical report of 93 cases. Chin Med J 82: 24–38, 1963.

19

Chemotherapy of Choriocarcinoma: Clinical and Fundamental Studies

Hiroyoshi Takamizawa, Souei Sekiya, Osamu Kobayashi, Hideo Matsui, and Tatsuya Oosaki

INTRODUCTION

Choriocarcinoma is a representative malignant tumor for which chemotherapy is the first choice of treatment [29]. Although it has not been clarified why choriocarcinoma responds well to chemotherapy, its biological characteristics such as allograft nature to the host, rapid growth potential, and abundant blood supply may contribute to response [30]. The prognosis of choriocarcinoma was remarkably improved by the introduction of methotrexate (MTX), actinomycin-D (Act-D) and triple MAC therapy (MTX, Act-D, and chlorambucil or cyclophosphamide [CPM]) [15]. However, approximately 40% of the patients with choriocarcinoma became refractory in spite of these intensive chemotherapies [29]. New protocols of chemotherapy, elucidation of drug resistance, and some new approaches are needed to improve the prognosis. We report here the efficacy and limitations of conventional chemotherapy against choriocarcinoma, clinical application of new combination chemotherapies designed by fundamental studies in vivo and in vitro, and different approaches to therapy.

MATERIALS AND METHODS

Patients

Included in the study were 371 patients with trophoblastic diseases that were diagnosed and treated in our Department during the 27 years from 1956 to 1983. These patients were histologically divided into three groups: invasive mole (115 cases), choriocarcinoma (88 cases), and histologically undetermined cases (168 cases). They were further divided into two groups by clinical risks since 1973: high-risk (53 cases) and low-risk (172 cases). High-risk was determined by the satisfaction of one of the following four criteria: 1) urinary human chorionic gonadotropin (U-hCG) titer over 100,000 IU/liter; 2) more than 1 year of an interval between the antecedent pregnancy and the initiation of therapy; 3) metastases to brain and/or liver; and 4) after full-term delivery. All patients with choriocarcinoma were included in the high-risk group, and 4 of 57 patients with invasive mole and 7 of 126 patients with undetermined cases were also included in the high-risk group.

Chemotherapy

The low-risk cases were treated with either MTX (20 mg intramuscularly, days 1 to 5) or Act-D (0.5 mg intravenously, days 1 to 5) alone or sequentially. The high-risk cases were initially treated with triple MAC combination therapy consisting of MTX (15 mg intramuscularly, days 1 to 5), Act-D (0.35 mg intravenously, days 1 to 5), and chlorambucil (8 mg orally, days 1 to 5) or CPM (100 mg intravenously, days 1 to 5). The patients who showed resistance to MAC therapy or had a relapse were treated with various modalities of combination chemotherapy.

Human Chorionic Gonadotropin Assay

A commercially available hemagglutination inhibition test (UCG titration, Kyorin Pharm. Co., Tokyo, Japan) or hemagglutination test (Hi-gonavis, Mochida Pharm. Co., Tokyo, Japan) was used to assay U-hCG. Serum (S)-hCG was assayed by CEA-IRE-SORIN hCG radioimmunoassay (RIA) kit (Green Cross Co., Osaka, Japan).

Determination of Remission

In low-risk patients, remission was determined when a patient showed a luteinizing hormone (LH) level of U-hCG by three consecutive weekly assays. In high-risk patients, it was determined when the U-hCG titers were within LH level for 3 months.

Nude Mice

Six- to seven-week-old female BALB/c nu/nu nude mice (Clea Japan Inc., Tokyo, Japan) were housed in barrier system. Two human choriocarcinoma strains, JCK and HM, that had been serially transplanted subcutaneously into nude mice were used for experimental chemotherapy [13]. The tumor tissues were minced with scissors into 1- to 2-mm^3 pieces and were transplanted subcutaneously into the femoral region of the nude mice. The drugs were given when the long diameter of tumor reached approximately 10 mm.

MTX (30 mg/kg), Act-D (0.032 mg/kg), CPM (100 mg/kg) and/or vincristine (VCR) (1 mg/kg) alone or in combination were administered every week into the peritoneal cavity of the nude mice. The animals were killed 3 days after the last administration and the tumors were resected. After measuring short (W) and long (L) diameters of tumor, the growth of tumor was calculated by $\frac{W^2 \times L}{2}$.

In Vitro Results

Eight kinds of human choriocarcinoma cell lines were used [23]. They were maintained by serial subcultivations in RPMI 1640 medium containing 10% newborn bovine serum at 37°C in a humidified 5% CO_2 incubator. For the estimation of ^3H-thymidine (6-

^{3}H-thymidine, 15 Ci/mmol, New England Nuclear Corp., Boston, Mass.) incorporation into cellular DNA, 10^5 cells in 1 mL of culture medium were seeded into a series of sterile scintillation vials. After 48 hours of incubation, the exponentially growing cells were exposed to MTX at doses from 10^{-9} to 10^{-4} M for 48 hours. Then ^{3}H-thymidine was added to each vial in 1 mL of culture medium at 1 μCi. After 30 minutes of incubation, each vial was quenched by the addition of 10 mL of ice-cold isotonic saline and the incorporation was counted with a scintillation counter, according to the method of Ball et al. [3]. For the estimation of cell growth, 10^5 cells were seeded into 60-mm plastic dishes (Becton Dickinson & Co., Oxnard, Calif.) in 5 mL of culture medium. After 48 hours, the culture medium was changed for that with or without 2×10^{-8} M MTX. The culture medium was then changed every other day for 8 days. The cells were detached from dishes with 0.25% trypsin solution, and viable cells were counted by the trypan blue dye exclusion test using a hemocytometer.

To isolate the MTX-resistant subline, the most MTX-sensitive HCCM-5 among the eight kinds of choriocarcinoma cell lines was fed with medium containing increasing concentrations of MTX [24, 25]. The initial MTX concentration, 10^{-9} M, which reduced the ^{3}H-thymidine incorporation, was raised from 2- to 2.5-fold successively. The isolation of MTX-resistant subline was followed for 80 weeks.

Pharmacokinetics of Methotrexate

Each of 10 patients was administered MTX by intravenous (450 mg) or intramuscular (20 mg) route. Serum MTX values were measured by an enzyme inhibition assay at various times (1 to 72 hours) after administration.

Tumor Angiogenesis Factor Activity

Four human choriocarcinoma cell lines were used to study tumor angiogenesis factor (TAF) activity. The growth in vitro was estimated by plating 10^5 cells as described above. Inoculation into hamster cheek pouches was done by injection of 2×10^6 cells into cortisone-conditioned 4-week-old female golden hamsters. Two to three animals per cell line were killed at 2 and 3 weeks after cell inoculation. The tumor tissues were resected, weighed, and fixed in 10% formalin. They were stained with hematoxylin and eosin for histologic examination and luxol fast-blue for examination of blood vessels.

Cell-free crude material of TAF was prepared by the modified method of Klagsbrun et al. [14]. The subconfluent cells in exponential growth were washed twice with lactate Ringer's medium. Approximately 10^7 cells in T-75 flasks were shaken at 4°C for 3 hours in 10 mL of lactate Ringer's solution. The solution was removed and centrifuged at $5{,}000 \times g$ for 10 minutes. The supernatant was then filtered through a 0.45-μm filter (Millipore Corp., Bedford, Mass.) and divided into 1 mL/vial. The samples were lyophilized and stored at −70°C until use. The lyophilized samples were dissolved in 100 μL of PBS solution and were soaked to the sterile 6-mm discs of Whatman GF/B glass fiber filters (Reeve-Angel, Clifton, N.J.), according to the method of Klagsbrun et al. [14]. The impregnanted filters with the supernatant of approximately 10^6 cells were put on the chorioallantoic membrane (CAM) of tenth day of the chick embryo, as described previously [26]. The angiogenic response of CAM to the samples was judged 3 days after inoculation. The CAM was excised carefully, photographed, and fixed in 10% formalin for histologic examination.

RESULTS

Clinical Results

During the 27 years from 1956 to 1983, 371 patients with trophoblastic disease were treated with chemotherapy in our Department. Table 1 demonstrates the remission rates of trophoblastic diseases by the year, chemotherapeutic drugs, and histologic diagnosis. An alkylating agent, nitrogen mustard, was not very effective against choriocarcinoma. The remission rate of choriocarcinoma was improved from 23% to 38% by employment of MTX or Act-D. With the introduction of triple MAC therapy in 1973, the remission rate has improved further, to 60%. At present, the remission rate for both invasive mole and undetermined cases is 100%.

Table 2 demonstrated the remission and recurrence rates by the clinical risk and histologic diagnosis in 225 cases since 1973, when an hCG RIA kit was first applied to assess remission. Recurrence was observed in 6 (24.0%) of 25 choriocarcinoma and in 3 (2.5%) of 119 undetermined cases, respectively. Thus the remission rate of the high-risk group with choriocarcinoma is not as high as expected.

We have tried various chemotherapy protocols for the recurrent cases after MAC therapy (Table 3). In addition to conventional chemotherapeutic drugs, VCR, bleomycin, cisplatin, and VP16-213 have been administered in various combinations. High-dose MTX with leucovorin rescue and Bagshawe's CHAMOMA protocol were also applied. However, the result was not satisfactory and no remission was obtained in 12 recurrent cases up to present (Table 3).

Table 1. Remission rate of 371 patients with trophoblastic disease (Chiba University, 1956–1983)

Period (agents)	Choriocarcinoma (%)	Invasive mole (%)	Undetermined (%)	Total (%)
1956–1963 (Alkylating agents)	5/22*(22.7)	31/38 (81.6)	0/2 (0)	36/62 (58.1)
1964–1972 (MTX or Act-D)	9/24 (37.5)	19/20 (95.0)	36/40 (90.0)	64/84 (76.2)
1973–1983 (Triple MAC therapy)†	25/42 (59.5)	57/57 (100)	126/126 (100)	208/225 (92.4)

Act-D=actinomycin-D; MAC=MTX, Act-D, and chlorambucil or cyclophosphamide; MTX=methotrexate.
* No. of remissions/no. of patients.
† Only to high-risk group (See Table 2).

Table 2. Remission and recurrence rates among 225 patients (Chiba University, 1973–1983)

Risk group	Histologic diagnosis	Remission rate (%)	Recurrence rate (%)
High	Choriocarcinoma	25/42* (59.5)	6/25† (24.0)
	Invasive mole	4/4 (100)	0/4 (0)
	Undetermined	7/6 (100)	0/7 (0)
Total		36/53 (67.9)	6/36 (16.7)
Low	Invasive mole	53/53 (100)	0/53 (0)
	Undetermined	119/119 (100)	3/119 (2.5)
Total		172/172 (100)	3/172 (1.7)

* No. of remissions/no. of patients.
† No. of recurrences/no. of remissions.

Table 3. Trial chemotherapy and results for cases resistant to MAC or recurrent cases

Chemotherapy	Case	Previous chemotherapy	Response	Prognosis
MTX+Act-D+CPM+VCR	W.A.	MAC	+	Remission
	H.M.	MAC	±	Death
CHAMOMA	T.T.	MAC	−	Death
	H.T.	MAC, CMA_3, ADM VCR, MPL	−	Death
	S.K.	MAC	+	Remission, recurrence
CPM+Act-D+VCR BLM, VP16-213	S.K.	CHAMOMA	−	Death
CDDP+BLM+VLB	Y.H.	MAC, VCR, CA	±	Death
	H.M.	VCR, ADM	−	Death
Ultrahigh dose MTX+CF	Y.H.	CDDP+BLM+VLB, CMA_3	−	Death
	H.M.	CDDP+BLM+VLB, ADM	−	Death
	H.T.	CHAMOMA, CMA_3, ADM, MPL	−	Death
Act-D+CPM	O.T.	MAC	+	Remission, recurrence

ADM=adriamycin; BLM=bleomycin; CDDP=cisplatin; CF=calcium leucovorin or citrovorum factor; CHAMOMA=HU, MTX+CF, VCR, Act-D, CPM, ADM, MPL; CMA_3=chromomycin A3; CPM=cyclophosphamide; HU=hydroxyuria; MPL=melphalan; VCR=vincristine; VLB=vinblastin. Other abbreviations as in Table 1.

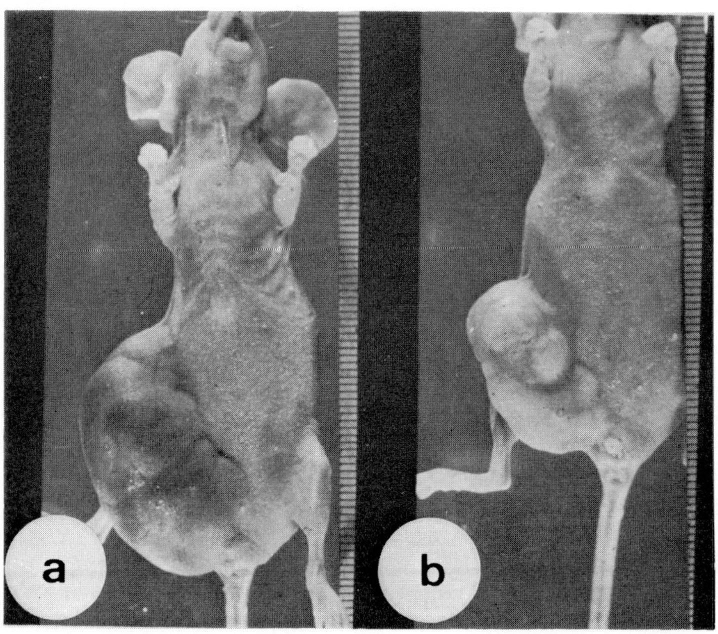

Figure 1. Xenografts of two human choriocarcinomas into nude mice. a=JCK; b=HM.

Fundamental Studies in Vivo and in Vitro

To establish more effective chemotherapy protocols, in vivo and in vitro studies using human choriocarcinomas were undertaken. Two different kinds of human choriocarcinoma strains, JCK and HM, that had been serially transplanted into nude mice were used. JCK was a rapidly growing tumor with mass lesions of bleeding and necrosis, whereas HM was a slowly growing tumor with solid whitish yellow mass (Figure 1). The effects of various combination chemotherapy protocols are demonstrated in Figure 2.

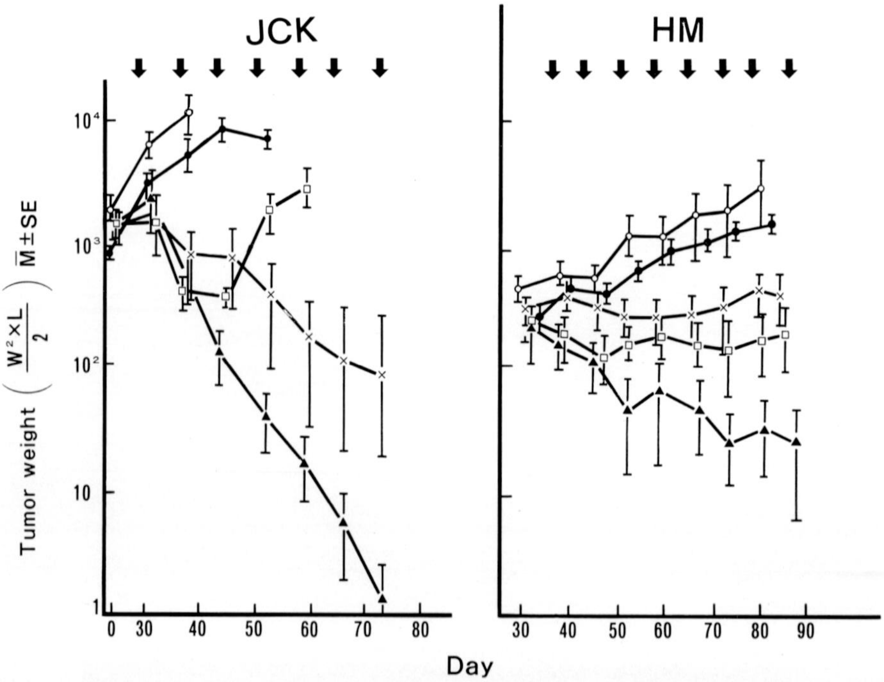

Figure 2. Experimental chemotherapies against the xenografts. ○=nontreated; ●=MTX+Act-D; □=MTX+CPM; ×=MTX+Act-D+CPM; ▲=MTX+VCR+Act-D; arrows= treatment.

The combination of MTX, VCR, and Act-D was the most effective against the two strains among the four combination protocols. The complete disappearance of tumor was observed in JCK, but it was less effective against HM.

In vitro experiments were then undertaken to elucidate the heterogeneity of sensitivity to human choriocarcinoma cells to chemotherapeutic drugs and process of drug resistance. Because it has been widely used and is considered one of the most effective drugs against trophoblastic disease, MTX was chosen as the chemotherapeutic agent. The inhibition of ^{3}H-thymidine incorporation of eight different kinds of human choriocarcinoma cell lines after 48 hours' culture in the medium containing MTX (from 10^{-9} to 10^{-4} M) and inhibition of growth in the medium containing 2×10^{-8} M were demonstrated in Figure 3. Such cell lines as HCCM-5, BeWo, and IMa showed sensitivity to MTX and their incorporation of ^{3}H-thymidine was suppressed by more than 10^{-8} M MTX. In parallel with the inhibition of ^{3}H-thymidine incorporation, their growth was also inhibited by 2×10^{-8} M and the inhibition became more prominent day by day. In contrast with these cell lines, both SCH and HM cell lines were completely resistant to MTX. Other cell lines such as JAr, JEG-3, and NUC-1 showed an intermediate sensitivity to MTX. Thus, a heterogeneity of sensitivity to MTX among these eight kinds of human choriocarcinoma cell lines was clearly demonstrated.

To examine the process of MTX resistance, we attempted to isolate a MTX-resistant subline from the most MTX-sensitive HCCM-5 cell line by increasing MTX concentration in the medium. The attempt was started from 10^{-9} M, and we obtained 36 weeks later a subline that grew normally in medium containing 5×10^{-7} M (Figure 4). However, we failed to establish a 10^{-6} M-resistant subline. This result may support the efficacy of high-dose MTX with citrovorum rescue in MTX-resistant choriocarcinoma.

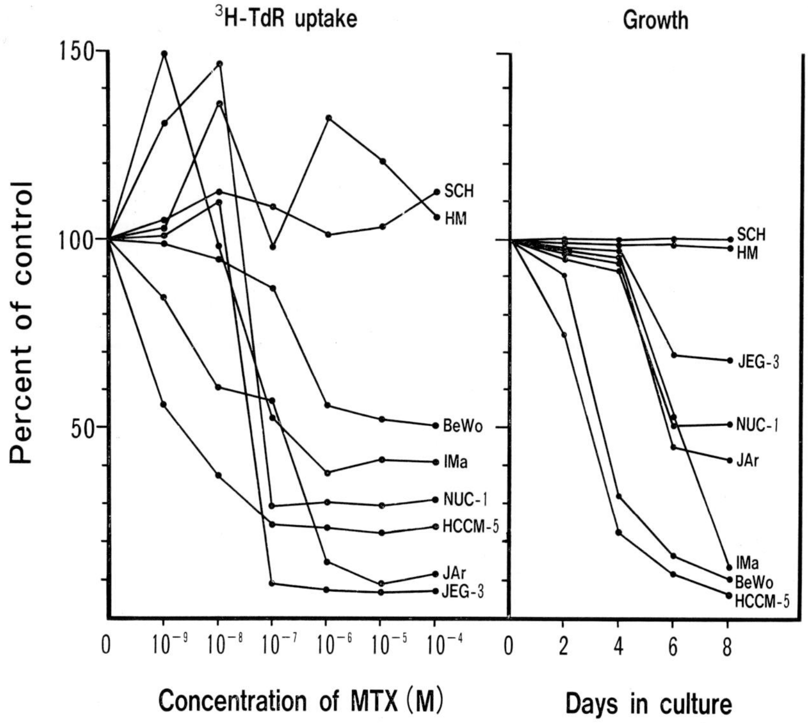

Figure 3. Effect of MTX on the inhibition of ^{3}H-thymidine uptake and growth of eight kinds of human choriocarcinoma cell lines in vitro. The growth inhibition was examined by continuous treatment of cells with 2×10^{-8} M.

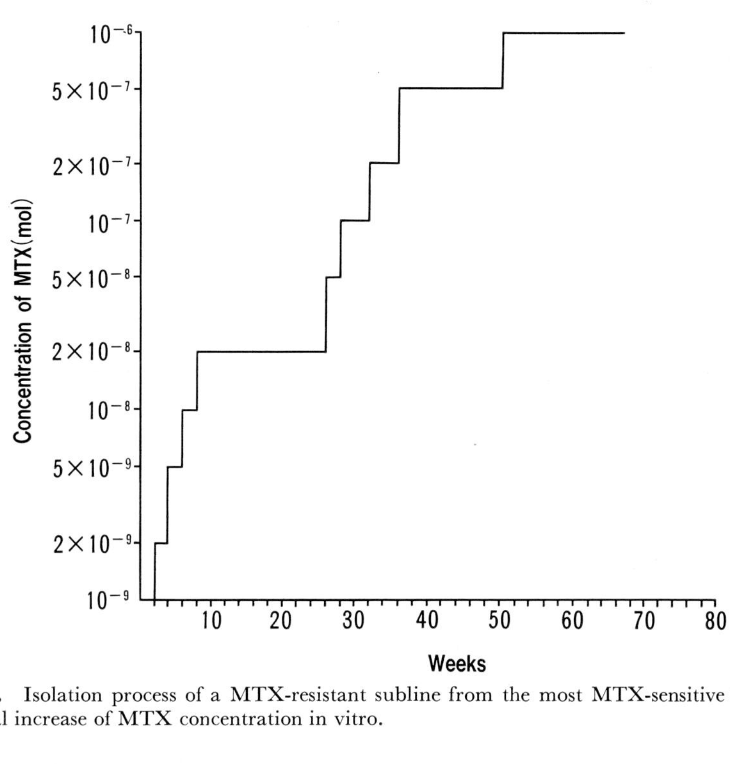

Figure 4. Isolation process of a MTX-resistant subline from the most MTX-sensitive HCCM-5 by gradual increase of MTX concentration in vitro.

Clinical Application: A New Protocol

Figure 5 demonstrates serum levels in patients who received 450 mg of MTX intravenously or 20 mg of MTX intramuscularly. In the former, serum MTX levels were found to reach 10^{-5} M. Taking into consideration the results obtained from these fundamental in vivo and in vitro studies and the pharmacokinetics of the chemotherapeutic drugs, a new combination protocol consisting of high-dose MTX, VCR, and Act-D (MOA therapy) has been brought to clinical practice. The protocol of MOA therapy is shown in Table 4. The MOA therapy has been applied to two relapse choriocarcinomas after MAC therapy and to three high-risk choriocarcinomas (Table 5). In particular, case O.T. experienced three relapses after intensive combination chemotherapies of MAC, cisplatin, and VP16-213. All of these patients achieved remission.

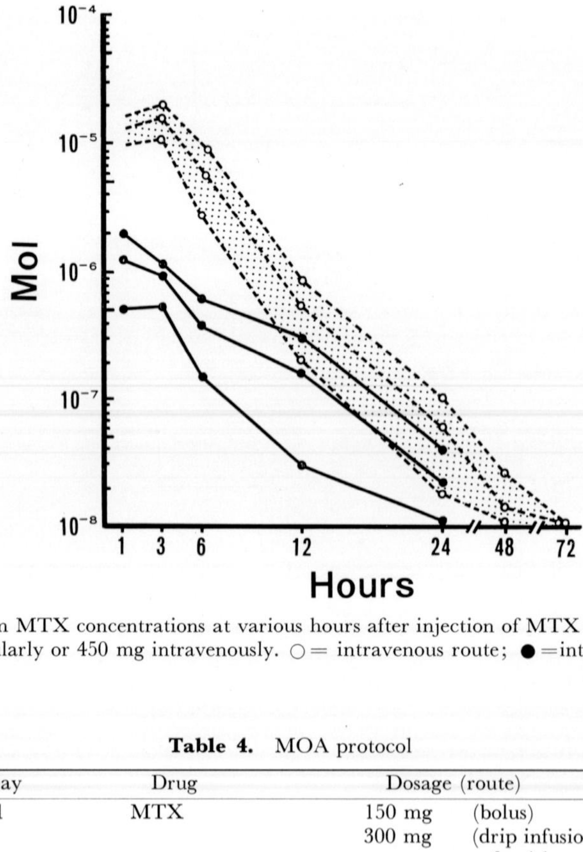

Figure 5. Serum MTX concentrations at various hours after injection of MTX by route of either 20 mg intramuscularly or 450 mg intravenously. ○ = intravenous route; ● = intramuscular route.

Table 4. MOA protocol

Day	Drug	Dosage (route)	
1	MTX	150 mg	(bolus)
		300 mg	(drip infusion for 4 hours)
	Oncovin	2 mg	(bolus)
	Act-D	0.5 mg	(bolus)
2	Act-D	0.5 mg	
	Leucovorin	15 mg (im) × 2	
3	Act-D	0.5 mg	
	Leucovorin	15 mg (im)	
4, 5	Act-D	0.5 mg	

im = intramuscularly.
Other abbreviations as in Table 1.

Table 5. Result of MOA protocol for choriocarcinoma

Case	Age (yr)	Antecedent pregnancy	Pretreatment hCG (IU/liter)	Metastasis	Previous chemotherapy	Response
O.T.	32	Full term	3,200	Lung	MAC, Act-D, CPM MTX+VCR+BLM+CDDP	CR
S.T.	49	H. mole	3,200	Lung	MAC	CR
Y.K.	38	Full term	102,400	(—)	(—)	CR
S.Y.	44	Full term	256,000	(—)	(—)	CR
S.S.	52	H. mole	25,600	(—)	(—)	CR

CR=complete remission; H. mole=hydatidiform mole.
Other abbreviations as in Tables 1 and 2.

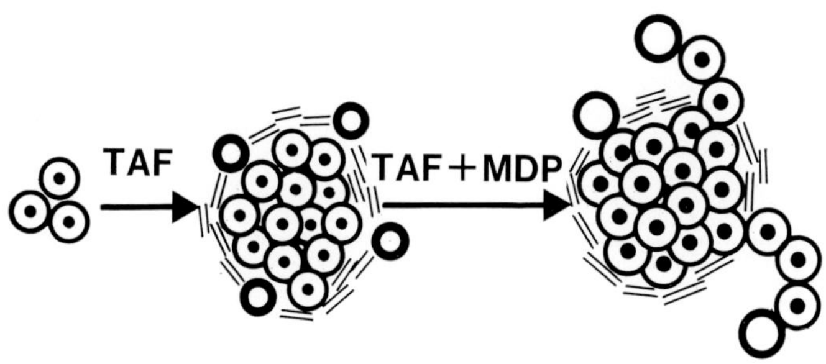

Figure 6. Possible mechanisms of growth, invasion, and metastasis of choriocarcinoma. TAF= tumor angiogenesis factor; MDP=matrix degrading proteinases.

A New Approach

Our experience in the treatment of choriocarcinoma with conventional surgery and chemotherapy seems to suggest a limitation of these therapies. Therefore, we are now trying new approach to therapy. Figure 6 is a schema explaining the possible mechanisms of the growth and metastasis of choriocarcinoma. Choriocarcinoma is a suitable model for this kind of study because it is a representative malignant tumor consisting of abundant blood vessels and showing rapid hematogenous metastasis. Neovascularization may be necessary for tumor growth. Choriocarcinoma cells may possibly secrete TAFs for their growth. In addition to TAF, matrix degrading proteinases (MDP) such as plasminogen activator, collagenase, and cathepsin B are also related to the tumor invasion and metastasis.

There was no significant difference among four cell lines in in vitro growth curves. However, among the cell lines implanted by xenograft into the hamster cheek pouches, a marked difference was observed in the growth curve. Rapidly growing tumors in vivo were found to be rich in vessels (Figure 7). These results suggest that the rapidly growing tumor cells in vivo secrete more TAF than slowly growing tumor cells.

The TAF activity of cell-free crude samples that were obtained by the supernatant of cultivated cells in lactate Ringer's medium was assayed using the CAM of chick embryos. Cell lines such as BeWo and JEG-3 that formed large tumors in vivo induced positive vascular response in high rate on the CAM, as compared with the cell lines such as SCH and HM, which showed slow growth in vivo (Figure 8). Purification of TAF is now being carried out. Purified TAF enables us to raise anti-TAF antibody or find specific antagonists to TAF. By the administration of these antagonists to TAF, angiogenesis might be inhibited, which may result in tumor regression.

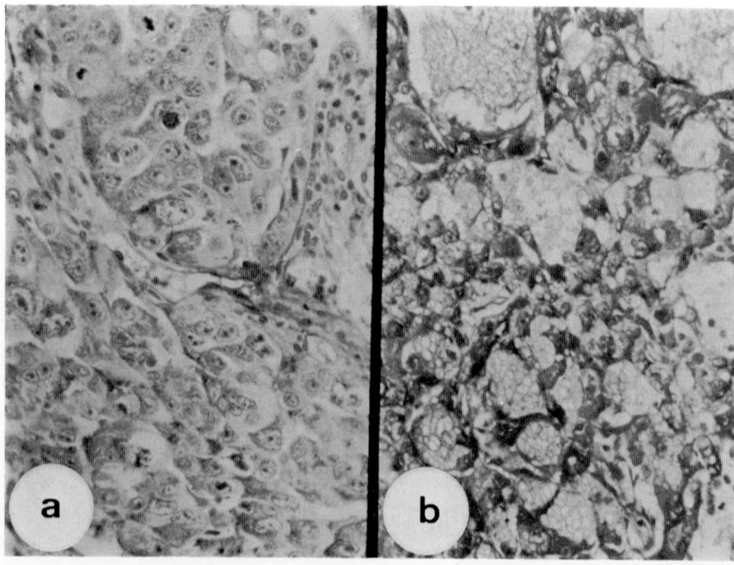

Figure 7. Xenografts of two human choriocarcinoma cell lines into hamster cheek pouches. a=SCH; b=BeWo. A large number of blood vessels are revealed in BeWo by luxol fast-blue stain. (Original magnification ×200.)

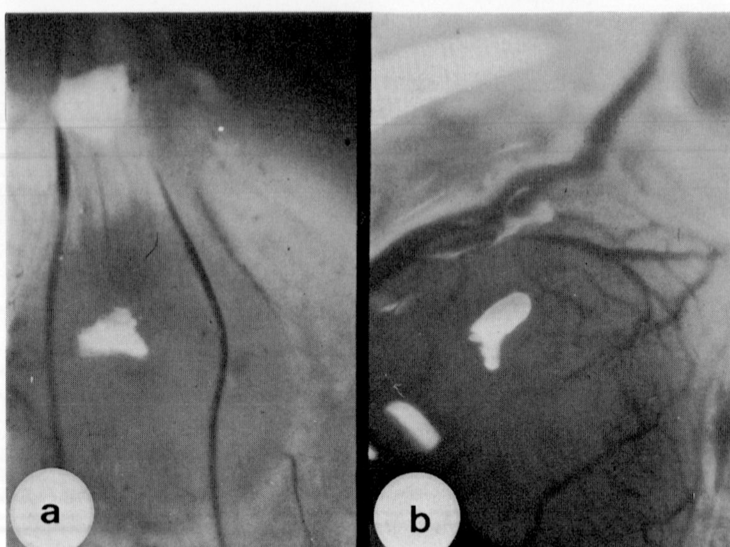

Figure 8. Vascular response in chorioallantoic membranes of the chick embryo. a=SCH; b=BeWo. Positive finding is observed in BeWo. (Original magnification ×10.)

DISCUSSION

The prognosis of choriocarcinoma was poor before introduction of MTX. The efficacy of MTX has become evident by several reports since 1956 [12, 16] and has remained as one of the most effective drugs [7, 27]. Next, Act-D was introduced, and it has been revealed that Act-D is useful in the treatment of patients with MTX-resistant choriocarcinoma [20, 21]. Further improvement of the prognosis has been accomplished by a combination triple MAC chemotherapy, consisting of MTX, Act-D and some alkylating agents [17]. In our studies, approximately 60% of choriocarcinoma cases have achieved remission since 1973. This remission rate is similar to that reported by other investigators [15].

Thus, choriocarcinoma has become one of the malignant tumors most sensitive to chemotherapeutic agents. Although it has not been clarified why choriocarcinoma responds well to chemotherapy, its biological characteristics such as allograft nature to the host, rapid growth potential, and abundant blood supply may contribute to good response [30].

Some prognostic factors of choriocarcinoma have been identified [1, 8, 11, 29]. All metastatic choriocarcinomas are included in the high-risk group of trophoblastic disease in our criteria. Almost all patients with invasive mole and histologically undetermined trophoblastic disease are included in the low-risk group, and they are curable by conventional chemotherapy modalities. Therefore, further development and introduction of new drugs and multiagents regimens are now urgently required to treat high-risk choriocarcinomas that shows resistance to conventional chemotherapy modalities. New protocols such as high-dose MTX with citrovorum factor rescue [4, 9, 32], various multiagents regimens by Bagshawe [2] and their modifications [28, 31], cisplatin in combination with VCR and MTX [18] or with VCR and bleomycin [10, 22] and VP16-213 [19] have been tried. Although remission has been obtained in sporadic cases, our results seem to be unsatisfactory.

Additional fundamental studies are required to improve the prognosis of these high-risk choriocarcinomas. At present, two experimental systems using human choriocarcinoma cells in vivo and in vitro are generally employed. Recently, intra- or intertumor heterogeneity has been considered to be a factor of drug resistance. Our fundamental studies using many kinds of human choriocarcinoma cell lines in vitro revealed that heterogeneity of sensitivity to MTX existed among the cell lines [24]. The heterogeneity was also noted in two xenografts of choriocarcinoma tissues in nude mice [13]. Another factor of drug resistance is acquired resistance in the course of chemotherapy. We revealed that the most MTX-sensitive cell line, HCCM-5, which was sensitive to 10^{-9} M, became resistant to 5×10^{-7} M within 36 weeks by gradual increases of the MTX concentration. The development of resistance was accompanied by both a decrease of the MTX uptake and an elevation of intracellular dihydrofolate reductase. Trial of isolation of a subline that showed resistance to more than 10^{-6} M was unsuccessful [25].

From the results obtained from these in vitro studies, experimental chemotherapy using the xenografts into nude mice, and pharmacokinetic studies on chemotherapeutic drugs in human, we developed a new combination protocol of chemotherapy. Although the cases have been too small to appreciate its efficacy, the MOA therapy consisting of high-dose MTX with citrovorum rescue, VCR, and Act-D induced remission in two high-risk choriocarcinomas that showed resistance to MAC therapy and other multidrug regimens.

Finally, distinct approaches from conventional therapeutic modalities are necessary for further improvement of the prognosis of choriocarcinoma. The malignant tumors need blood supply for their progressive growth in the host. It has been demonstrated that the malignant tumor cells produce and secrete factors that induce new blood vessels from the surrounding host tissue [6]. Choriocarcinoma seems to be an ideal model of neovascularization because it is a representative tumor that contains abundant blood vessels. Ehrmann and Knoth [5] reported that choriocarcinoma tissues transplanted into hamster cheek pouch produced and secreted factors that could stimulate the proliferation of new blood vessels. The TAFs detected in the culture medium of our human choriocarcinoma cell lines also formed large tumors in hamster cheek pouch. If the purified TAF is obtained, anti-TAF antibody or specific antagonists to TAF may be selected, and they may be useful for the diagnosis and treatment of choriocarcinoma.

SUMMARY

In our study, approximately 60% of choriocarcinoma cases achieved remission since 1973 by treatment with conventional chemotherapies, consisting chiefly of MAC protocol. At present, further development and introduction of new drugs and multiagents regimens are urgently required to treat the high-risk choriocarcinomas resistant to conventional chemotherapy modalities. Although several new protocols showed efficacy in sporadic cases, the results have been unsatisfactory. We developed new protocol consisting of high-dose MTX with citrovorum rescue, VCR, and Act-D (MOA therapy) from the results obtained from in vitro studies, experimental chemotherapy using xenografts into nude mice, and the pharmocokinetics of the drugs in humans. This protocol has been effective in five choriocarcinomas, including two drug-resistant cases. Finally, a distinct approach to the therapy based on neovascularization by TAF is suggested.

REFERENCES

1. Bagshawe KD: Risk and prognostic factors in trophoblastic neoplasia. Cancer 38: 1373–1375, 1976.
2. Bagshawe KD: Treatment of high-risk choriocarcinoma. J Reprod Med 29: 813–820, 1984.
3. Ball CR, Roynter RW, van den Berg HW: A novel method for measuring incorporation of radioactive precursors into nucleic acid and proteins of cells in monolayer culture. Anal Biochem 46: 101–107, 1972.
4. Berkowitz RS, Goldstein DP, Jones MA, Marean AR, Bernstein MR: Methotrexate with citrovorum factor rescue. Reduced chemotherapy toxicity in the management of gestational trophoblastic neoplasms. Cancer 45: 423–426, 1980.
5. Ehrmann RL, Knoth M: Choriocarcinoma: Transfilter stimulation of vasoproliferation in the hamster cheek pouch—study by light and electron microscopy. J Natl Cancer Inst 41: 1329–1341, 1968.
6. Folkman J, Costran R: Relation of vascular proliferation to tumor growth. Int Rev Exp Pathol 16: 207–248, 1976.
7. Freedman RS: Methotrexate in gestational trophoblastic disease. Cancer Bull 33: 63–66, 1981.
8. Goldstein DP: The chemotherapy of gestational trophoblastic disease. Principles of clinical management. JAMA 220: 209–213, 1972.
9. Goldstein DP, Saracco P, Osathanondh R, Goldstein PR, Marean AP, Bernstein MR: Methotrexate with citrovorum factor rescue for gestational trophoblastic neoplasms. Obstet Gynecol 51: 93–96, 1978.
10. Hainsworth JD, Burnett LS, Jones HW III, Greco FA: Resistant gestational choriocarcinoma: Successful treatment with vinblastine, bleomycin, and cisplatin (VBP). Cancer Treat Rep 67: 393–395, 1983.
11. Hammond CB, Borchert LG, Tyrey LK, Creasman W, Parker RT: Treatment of metastatic trophoblastic disease: Good and poor prognosis. Am J Obstet Gynecol 115: 451–457, 1973.
12. Hertz R, Lewis J Jr, Lipsett MB: Five years' experience with the chemotherapy of metastatic choriocarcinoma and related trophoblastic tumors in women. Am J Obstet Gynecol 82: 631–640, 1961.
13. Katoh T, Ishige H, Kobayashi O, Takamizawa H, Tokita H, Tanaka N: Experimental chemotherapy with human choriocarcinoma transplanted in nude mice and the clinical application (in Japanese). Gan To Kagaku Ryoho 8: 1974–1981, 1981.
14. Klagsbrun M, Knighton D, Folkman J: Tumor angiogenesis activity in cells grown in tissue culture. Cancer Res 36: 110–114, 1976.
15. Lewis JL Jr: Treatment of metastatic gestational trophoblastic neoplasms. A brief review of developments in the years 1968 to 1978. Am J Obstet Gynecol 136: 163–172, 1980.
16. Li MC, Hertz R, Spencer DR: Effects of methotrexate therapy upon choriocarcinoma. Proc Soc Exp Biol Med 93: 361–366, 1956.

17. Li MC: Management of choriocarcinoma and related tumors of uterus and testis. Med Clin North Am 45: 661–676, 1961.
18. Newlands ES, Bagshawe KD: Activity of high-dose *cis*-platinum (NUI 119875) in combination with vincristine and methotrexate in drug-resistant gestational choriocarcinoma. A report of 17 cases. Br J Cancer 40: 943–945, 1979.
19. Newlands ES, Bagshawe KD: The role of VP 16–213 (etoposide; NSC-141540) in gestational choriocarcinoma. Cancer Chemother Pharmacol 7: 211–214, 1982.
20. Ross GT, Stolbach LL, Hertz R: Actinomycin D in the treatment of methotrexate-resistant trophoblastic disease in women. Cancer 22: 1015–1017, 1962.
21. Ross GT, Goldstein DP, Hertz R, Lipsett MB, Odell WD: Sequential use of methotrexate and actinomycin D in the treatment of metastatic choriocarcinoma and related trophoblastic diseases in women. Am J Obstet Gynecol 93: 223–229, 1965.
22. Schlaerth JB, Morrow CP, DePetrillo AD: Sustained remission of choriocarcinoma with cis-platinum, vinblastine, and bleomycin after failure of conventional combination drug therapy. Am J Obstet Gynecol 136: 983–985, 1980.
23. Sekiya S, Shirotake S, Kaiho T, Iwasawa H, Kawata M, Higaki K, Ishige H, Takamizawa H, Minamihisamatsu M: A newly established human gestational choriocarcinoma cell line and its characterization. Gynecol Oncol 15: 413–421, 1983.
24. Sekiya S, Kaiho T, Shirotake S, Iwasawa H, Takeda B, Takamizawa H: Effect of methotrexate on the growth and human chorionic gonadotropin secretion of human choriocarcinoma cell lines in vitro. Am J Obstet Gynecol 146: 57–64, 1983.
25. Sekiya S, Kaiho T, Takamizawa H: Development of methotrexate-resistant human choriocarcinoma cells in culture. Gynecol Oncol 21: 46–53, 1985.
26. Sekiya S, Oosaki T, Suzuki N, Takamizawa H: Invasive potential of human choriocarcinoma cell lines and the role of lytic enzymes. Gynecol Oncol (in press).
27. Sobrero A, Bertino JR: The role of methotrexate in the chemotherapy of gestational trophoblastic neoplasms. In Pattillo RA, Hussa RO (eds): Human Trophoblast Neoplasms. Plenum, New York, 1984, pp. 343–354.
28. Surwit EA, Suciu TN, Schmidt HJ, Hammond CB: A new combination chemotherapy for resistant trophoblastic disease. Gynecol Oncol 8: 110–118, 1979.
29. Takamizawa H, Katoh T, Sekiya S, Endoh N, Kikuchi Y, Kudoh J: The prognostic factors of the "high risk" trophoblastic neoplasia. In Thatcher N (ed): Advances in Medical Research and Education, Vol. 8: Gynecological Cancer. Pergamon, Elmsford, NY, 1979, pp. 271–279.
30. Takamizawa H, Sekiya S: Cell biology of choriocarcinoma. A brief review. Asia Oceania J Obstet Gynaecol 10: 245–256, 1984.
31. Weed JC Jr, Barnard DE, Currie JL, Clayton LA, Hammond CB: Chemotherapy with the modified Bagshawe protocol for poor prognosis metastatic trophoblastic disease. Obstet Gynecol 59: 377–380, 1982.
32. Wong LC, Choo YC, Ma HK: Methotrexate with citrovorum factor rescue in gestational trophoblastic disease. Am J Obstet Gynecol 152: 59–62, 1985.

Index

E

F

G

H

I

K

L

M

N

O

P

Q

R

S

T

V

W

X

Y

Z